EAST RENFREWSHIRE
09398260

KT-417-237

eat smart

NIOMI SMART

This book is dedicated to you.

You, who have been there since day one and who have followed me on my journey every step of the way, and you, who have picked up this book and decided to give me a chance.

Without you I wouldn't be where I am today. I am lucky to have subscribers, followers, readers and friends, and I couldn't be happier that you are one of them.

Thank you for listening to me, trying my recipes and hopefully being inspired.

Thank you for making this book possible.

Niomi

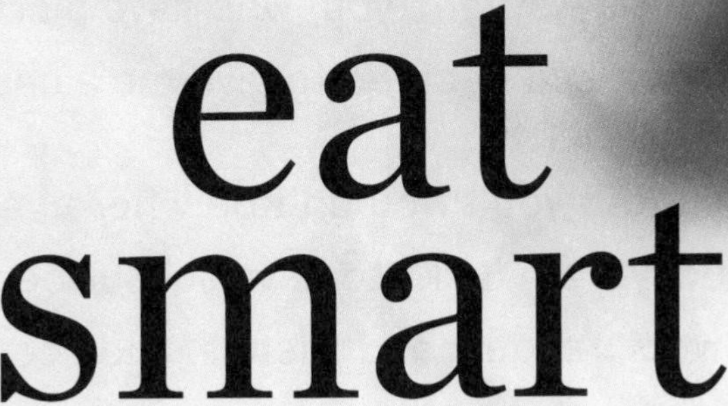

what to eat in a day – every day

NIOMI SMART

HarperCollins*Publishers*

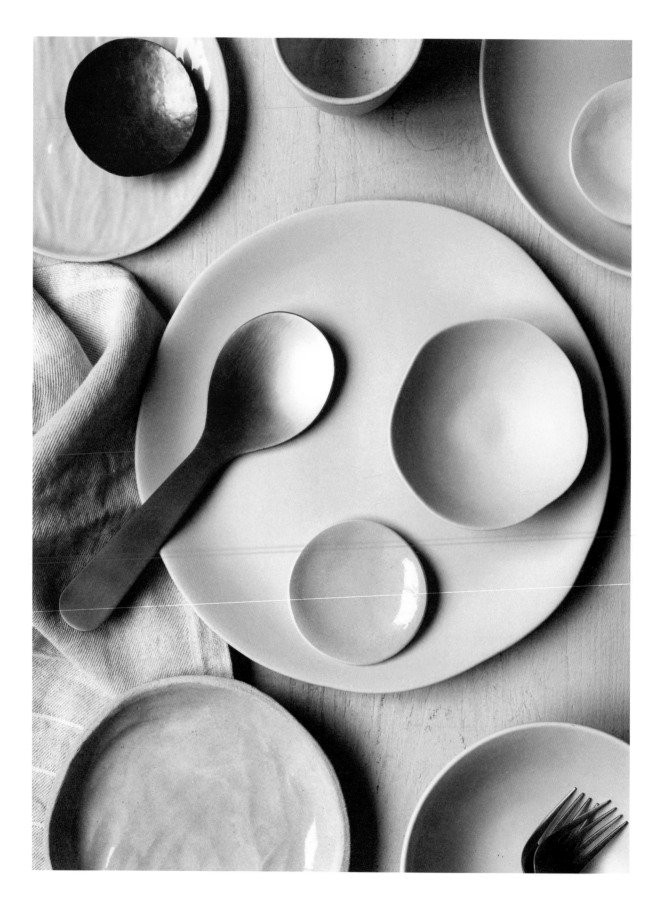

CONTENTS

WELCOME

Welcome to *Eat Smart*! I'm Niomi Smart, a lifestyle blogger and co-founder of the healthy snack boxes SourcedBox. After transitioning to a plant-based diet in 2014, I started to create my own recipes and share them with my audience on my Instagram, YouTube channel and blog. Some of my most popular videos have been my 'What I Eat in a Day' series, where I showcase all the delicious meals I have throughout the day. This has inspired the structure of *Eat Smart*. People seemed to really enjoy them and kept asking me for more, so I set myself a goal to write my own recipe book.

One thing you should know before we get started is that *Eat Smart* is in no way a diet book; it's a healthy cookbook and contains delicious recipes, all made from natural ingredients that do wonders for your health. Rather than putting you on a fad diet and restricting your food options, this book will help you learn to love your fresh fruit and vegetables and find easy, accessible recipes that you can incorporate into your busy life.

If you, like me, really notice the benefits of eating this way, you may find yourself also adopting a fully plant-based way of eating, or you may be happy with your overall diet but simply wish to include one or two plant-based healthy meals during the week. For whatever reason you picked up this book, I truly hope you enjoy every recipe and can tell how much thought and love I have put into it.

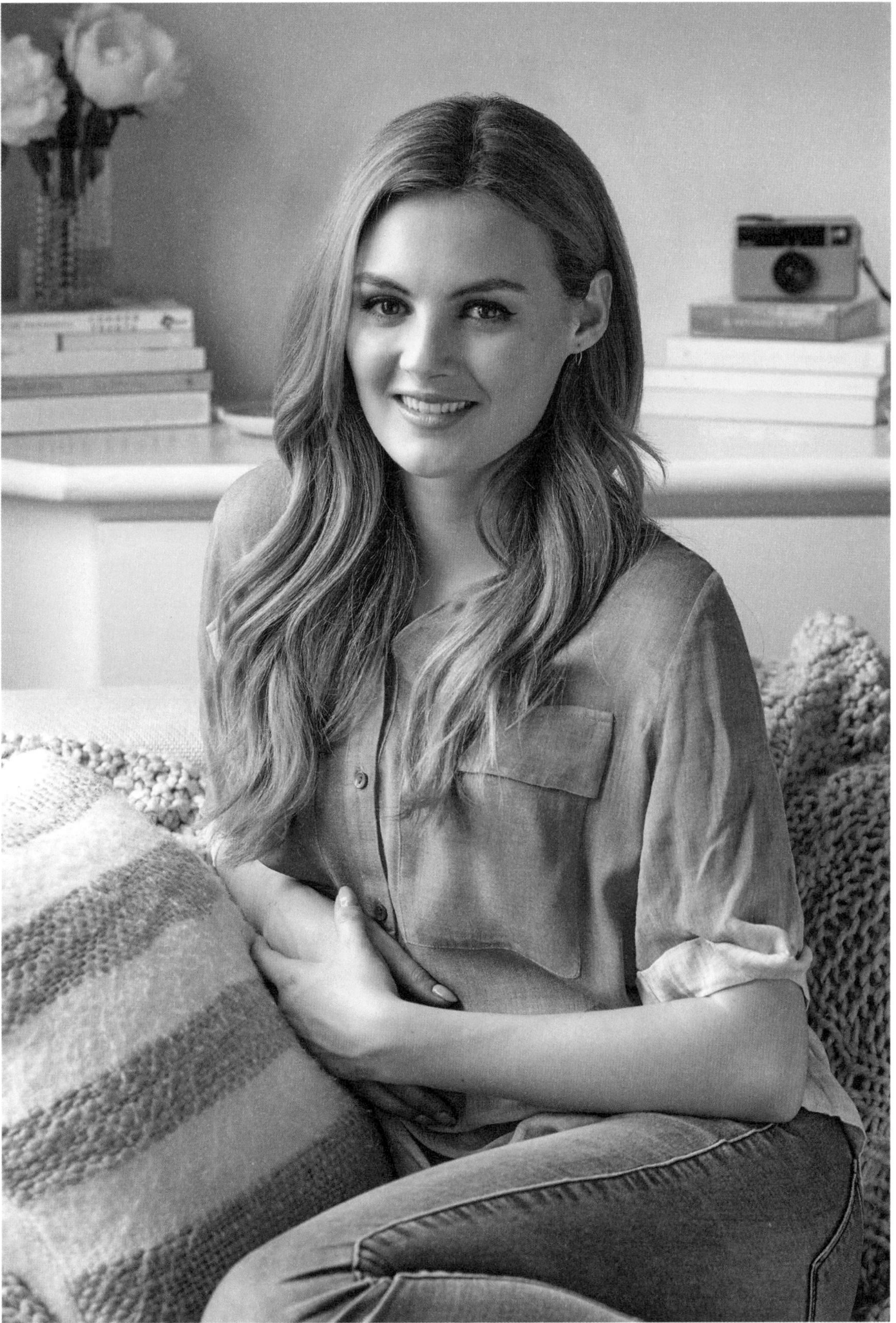

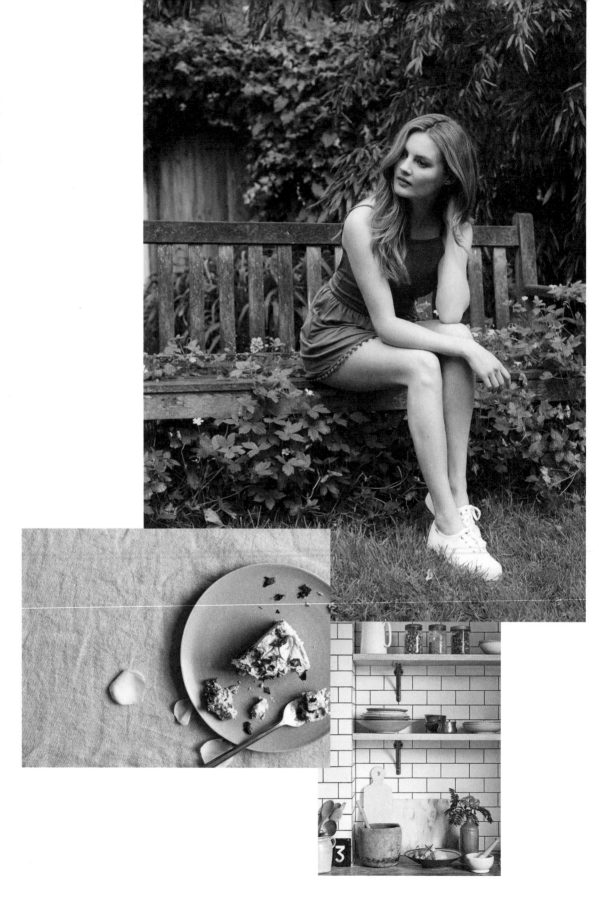
3

ABOUT ME

In 2010 I went to university to study Law, intending to pursue a career as a solicitor. I loved studying the legal system, but I realised near the end of my final year that practising Law was a whole other story and that this path wasn't for me. When I graduated it was a period of feeling proud and having a huge sense of accomplishment after years of hard work. Yet, at the same time I felt a sense of fear that I was now released into the adult world and expected to skip down the perfectly clear, yellow brick road that was my career, when actually it wasn't what I wanted. I created a blog in 2013, a couple of months after I graduated, because I found I had so many different passions outside of my law degree that I needed to have my own outlet where I could express myself in other ways, mainly focusing on beauty and fashion.

It was when I transitioned to a plant-based way of eating that my love of cooking really kicked off

After a few months I decided to also start my YouTube channel, where I could really connect with my audience that had grown on my blog. It was around this time that I discovered the importance of eating well, and that's when I found I was most passionate about making videos about health and wellbeing. I realised that healthy food doesn't have to be bland, and can in fact be fun and creative.

I would often Instagram my food and people would ask for the recipes, and that's when my 'What I Eat in a Day' videos were born. These videos range from what I eat when I'm travelling in places such as Bali, to what I eat when I'm training for a marathon in London. Hearing from people how they have been inspired by these videos and that they have had such a huge impact is incredibly rewarding and gives the videos a real purpose.

MY HEALTH JOURNEY

When I was younger, I never cooked at all. My grandma and mum have always been good cooks but I was never interested. I actually remember once telling them I would never cook, and that I'd just have to find a partner when I was older who could do it for me. Whenever I went to my grandparents' house after school, my grandma would sit me on the stool in the kitchen while she made dinner. I'd sit and chat to her, catching up on each other's days, and didn't realise that I was subconsciously learning what she was doing – she now admits to doing this for that exact purpose! For some reason cooking seemed a waste of time and boring, but then a few years ago I realised how important it was to prepare nutritious, homemade meals using fresh ingredients, and what an impact it would have on my overall wellbeing.

I want to inspire others to feel good by cooking food to nourish the body

Around the time that I started to look into a healthier way of living a couple of people in my life were diagnosed with serious illnesses, one of whom didn't make it. Fortunately for me it wasn't a direct family member, but the pain and hurt I saw in their relatives made me realise just how delicate life is. It made me question the food we have become accustomed to eating now – fast and processed, pumped full of sugar, salt, additives and all kinds of chemicals that are difficult to digest (mentally and physically), and it made me wonder what sort of an effect these foods have on our bodies. I started researching this and I couldn't believe how detrimental it can be to your health to eat this way. I decided to cut out processed foods and started to cook my own meals at home instead of buying ready meals, which was great, but I was still eating meat, fish, dairy and eggs. However, while doing my research the plant-based way of eating seemed to be a recurring topic.

Like many others, I had hugely misinterpreted eating plant-based as being restricted to bland salads lacking in flavour or substance. Unfortunately the word 'vegan' has a stigma attached to it. People picture 'vegans' looking pale and ill and being incredibly preachy about the way they eat. Some people may also think it's virtually impossible to eat this way because you will run out of things to eat, or the food simply doesn't taste as good. However, I decided to look into it more and noticed how appealing plant-based eating sounded, but then I'm a pretty open-minded person and love discovering new things, asking hundreds of questions of interesting people and finding out why they have made certain choices in life.

The more research I did, the more fascinating I found it hearing how much of a positive impact plant-based eating was having on people around the world, from supposedly curing illnesses to simply having more energy. I knew I couldn't come to my own decision until I tried it myself, so that's when I cut out all meat, fish, dairy and eggs from my diet overnight to see how it made me feel.

I had no idea how long I would eat this way because I decided to listen to my body rather than limiting myself to a set time scale. After only a couple of weeks of eating plant-based, I couldn't believe how different I felt. I had so much more energy, my skin looked clearer and brighter than ever, my hair and nails were growing at the speed of lightning and I felt happier and more positive. Since that day, over two years ago, I haven't looked back, which is why I wanted to create this recipe book.

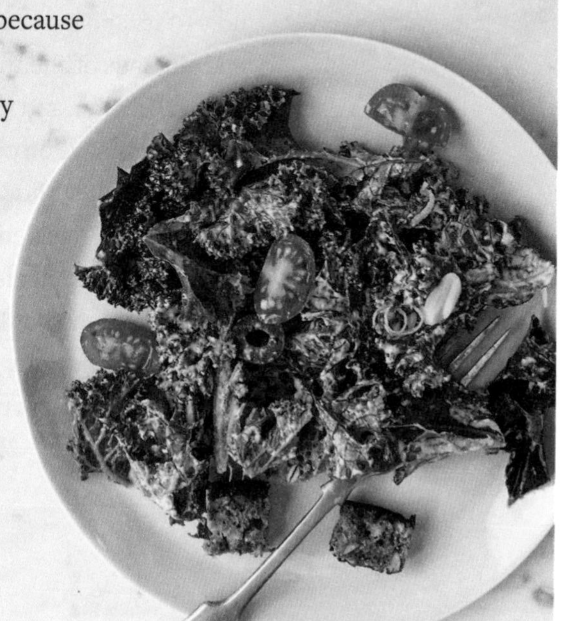

THE PLANT-BASED LIFESTYLE

This way of eating is all about embracing a lifestyle that may be quite different to what you're used to. I call this lifestyle plant-based, not vegan, because vegan refers to a diet and lifestyle that eliminates all animal products altogether – including honey – while a plant-based diet eliminates food products that come from animals, but can include honey, which I do eat occasionally provided it's locally and ethically sourced.

I never count calories. I think it's far more important to eat when you're hungry and stop eating when you're full, and to try to eat an abundance of whole foods

I chose to make a dramatic change to the way I ate overnight, but if I were to do it again I would take it step by step, to make it easier to adjust to all the changes. The prospect of a plant-based diet can seem daunting at first, because you focus on the things you have to cut out rather than the amazing things that you'll be introducing. So take small steps for a few weeks until you reach a point where you feel really happy. You don't have to go completely plant-based. I believe the way you eat is subjective because only you know what truly works for your own body. This way of eating suits me well, but it won't appeal to everyone, so try it, listen to your body and find the right balance. The main thing is to avoid processed foods and eat more fresh produce whenever you can.

The main motivator for me is knowing that I'm looking after myself, keeping myself healthy and respecting my body. One thing I should also mention is that I honestly couldn't tell you what my daily calorie intake is because I'm just not interested. For me, eating well isn't about restricting yourself to a specific calorie intake. For instance, nuts, avocados and coconuts are high in calories but their amazing health benefits outweigh the high calories.

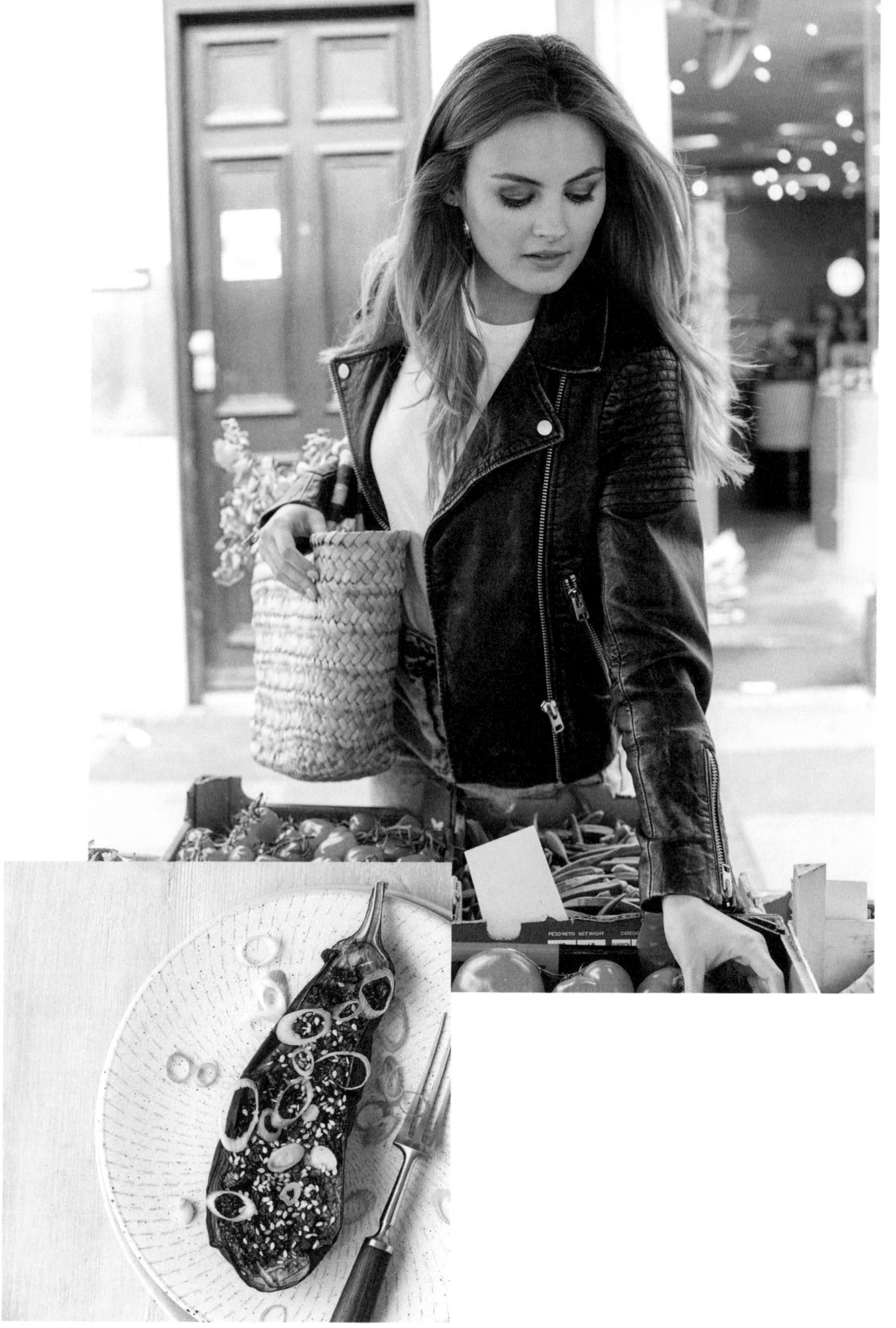

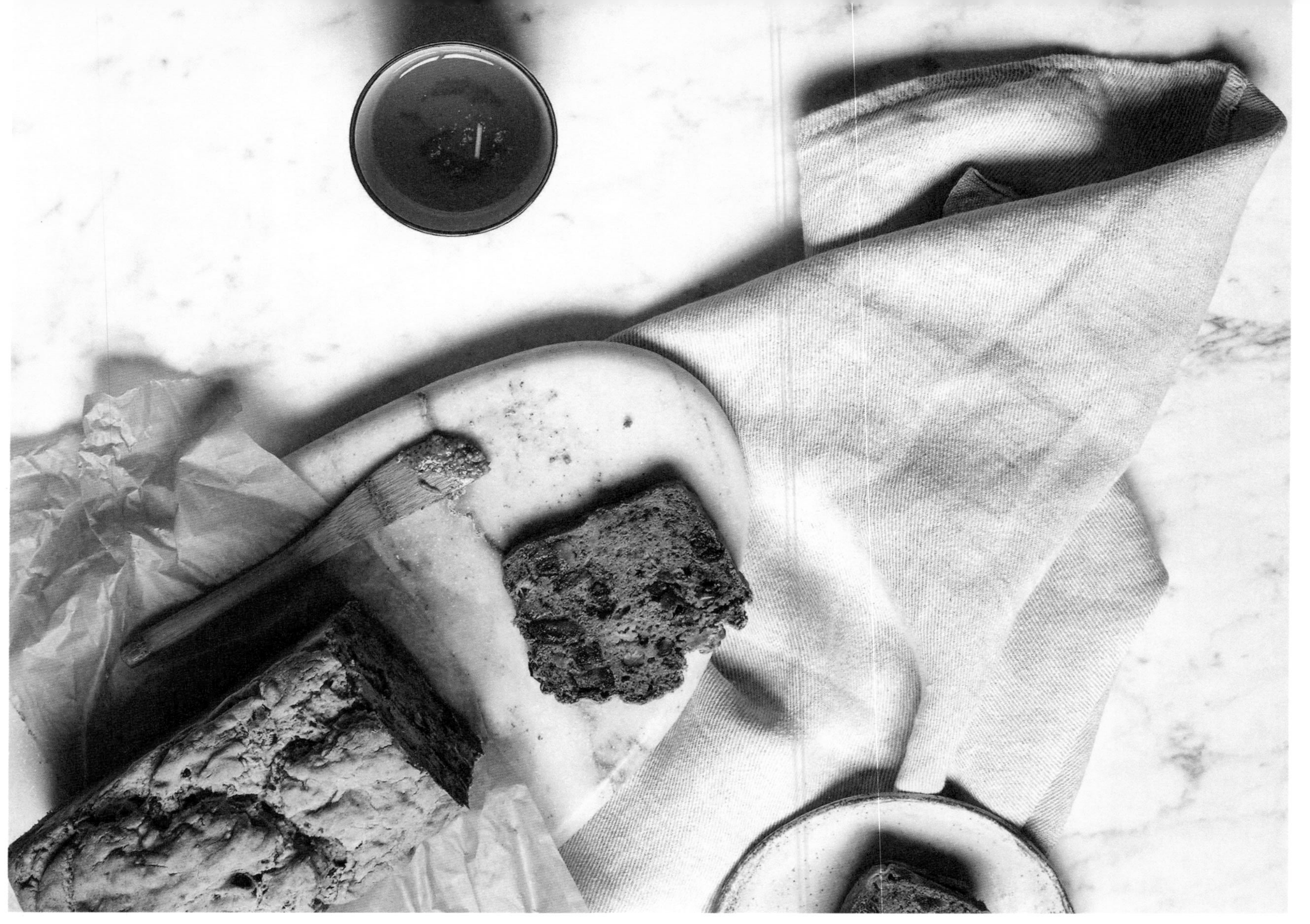

MY INSPIRATION

Due to my flexible job on YouTube, I'm lucky to have travelled to many different countries over the past few years and experienced various cultures and food. Many of my recipes have been inspired by the meals I have eaten while travelling, but they are created here with my own touch. I've adapted these authentic cooking methods to make the recipes easy and accessible, and always I use fresh ingredients, keeping health at the forefront of my mind.

My first experience of Asia was on a trip to Bali in 2015. The people were so friendly, happy and accommodating – I learnt a lot about the food there, particularly when one local invited me into their home and talked me through their typical daily meals. The Balinese really value the importance of eating well to nurture themselves for overall health, wellbeing and spirituality. A local told me how when they get sick they often heal themselves first through food and herbs before going to a conventional doctor. I, too, try to avoid over-the-counter medication wherever I can and, touch wood, since eating this way I have rarely become ill, but when I feel a cold or flu coming on, I nourish myself with natural food and spices such as ginger, oranges and turmeric.

Travelling has opened my eyes to different ingredients and encouraged me not to be scared of experimenting with food. The people that I meet all over the world really cement in my mind my views on health and wellbeing, but there are also people online that I have never met but who have had a big impact on my views, including Brendan Brazier, who created the Vega brand, and Matt Frazier, of the No Meat Athlete blog, whose podcasts I listen to while running.

CHANGING THE WAY YOU EAT

The hardest thing about changing the way you eat is most definitely the social aspect. Your friends and family may not approve of you eating healthier at first, which sounds crazy, right? Being healthily has a stigma attached to it – people can often think those who eat healthily are obsessive and self-obsessed. But this isn't always the case. When I first gave up meat, eggs and dairy many people were actually worried about my health, which baffled me because I was doing it for the opposite reason.

Another obstacle to overcome when you change the way you eat is finding places to eat out. Although many people have certain dietary requirements, it can still be tricky finding places that have something suitable on the menu. However, to this day, I have never had to leave a cafe or restaurant because they have nothing for me. I used to be embarrassed explaining to restaurant staff that I ate a plant-based diet, especially with people that I didn't know too well, but now I have realised that if you don't say anything, you're just going to be stuck with the one thing that's vegan on the menu – most likely a plain side salad. Eating this way is a positive and nothing to be embarrased by. You'd be surprised by how many people are interested and may be inspired.

Preparation is key. I cook more than I will eat in the evenings so that I have plenty of leftovers for lunch the next day – and food often tastes even better the next day because the flavours intensify overnight. Weekends are a great opportunity to make healthy snacks, such as energy balls (see page 168) for the week ahead. I'm such a grazer, so I like to have my handbag well stocked with healthy snacks and drinks. SourcedBox has been an amazing way to always have healthy snacks on the go.

An important aspect of any change in the way you eat is to be sure that you will not be lacking any vital vitamins and minerals. I've made sure that the *Eat Smart* recipes include foods naturally high in vitamins and minerals, but on a plant-based diet, the vitamins and minerals you may need to be more aware of are vitamin B12, calcium, iron and vitamin D, as well as omega-3 and protein.

There are so many natural plant-based sources of protein, though, such as peas, nuts, black beans, lentils and quinoa. I also occasionally add a vegan protein powder to my smoothies.

Calcium can be easily obtained from sources such as kale, chickpeas and black strap molasses, and you can get sufficient amounts of iron through wholegrains, lentils, chickpeas and black strap molasses again. To get a healthy amount of omega-3, include walnuts, chia seeds and flaxseed in your diet. You can also find non-dairy milks that are fortified with certain vitamins, too.

Fitting healthy eating into a busy lifestyle isn't as hard as you think

The two supplements that I take are B12 and vitamin D. Vitamin D can be gained purely from the sunlight, but unfortunately that's not so common here in the UK! You can also get vitamin D from mushrooms, but they have to be UV treated, and it can be hard to know that for sure. A lack of vitamin B12 can cause serious health problems, so it's one to be aware of. Even though B12 itself is a vegan product, it can be hard to get it eating only plant-based food. The best way to get B12 is to take a supplement – either as a capsule, tongue spray, injection or sublingual tablets. Sublingual tablets are small and sweet-tasting and can be placed under your tongue until they dissolve – this is the most effective way of getting B12 into your body because it doesn't have to go through the digestive system.

EXERCISE

At school I was never one of the naturally sporty kids, but I did enjoy a select few sports, such as cross-country running, rounders and netball. For any other sports I would come up with a million and one excuses to get out of them. Since becoming aware of the importance of eating well I have also taken up exercising; the two go hand in hand. Fortunately I now really enjoy working out and keeping fit, I love that feeling you have for the rest of the day after exercise.

I tend to work out three to five times a week and always mix up the sessions. My favourite workout is running because it gets your heart rate up, which is obviously the best thing for your cardiovascular health. I only run outdoors rather than in a gym because I find it more mentally stimulating, meaning I can run further and have got to know London better.

I also love strength training using weights or my own body weight to tone up. I find it motivating to see the changes in your body and to notice how much stronger you feel in yourself. I do yoga once a week to stretch out my muscles, especially as I do so much running, which has quite a high impact on the joints and muscles. It's important to include a lower-intensity workout if you're exercising a lot, and yoga is my favourite choice for this down time to relax and clear my mind.

I'm an early bird and have more energy at the start of the day, so I have always preferred to get active in the morning. If you need a little motivation to go to the gym in the morning, here's a tip: lay out your trainers and workout clothing and make one of my overnight breakfasts the night before, so you can throw on the gear and grab your breakfast as soon as you wake up and get straight to the gym without even thinking about it!

Many people think that eating plant-based wouldn't provide as much energy or muscle growth as a standard diet, but actually it is quite the opposite. I've never felt more energetic or fitter, and it fuelled me to run the London Marathon, which is a staggering 26.2 miles. The marathon was not something I'd thought about before but when I was approached by a charity to run it for them I of course took up the opportunity. I am convinced that had I not been eating the way I do now, I wouldn't have enjoyed it as much and most definitely would have struggled.

Exercise makes me feel great physically and psychologically and sets me up for the rest of the day, feeling positive, upbeat and generally happier

A lot of what I eat in a day depends on how much energy I'll be using, so if I'm doing an intense workout I'll focus on getting more carbohydrates and eat what my body is telling me it needs. On rest days where I do no exercise I lower my intake of carbohydrates because my body just doesn't need that extra energy. When I'm craving something filling and satisfying I'll opt for something higher in fat, such as almond butter.

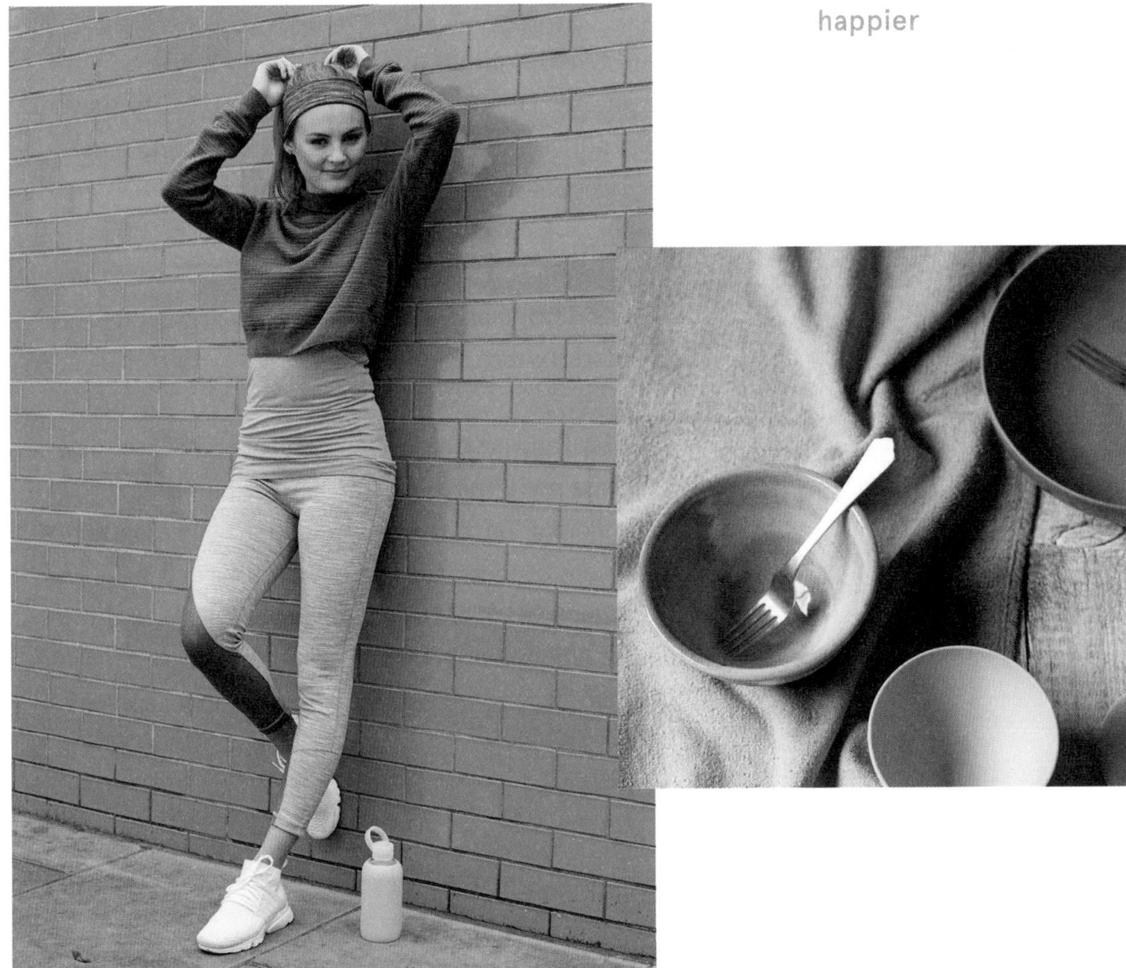

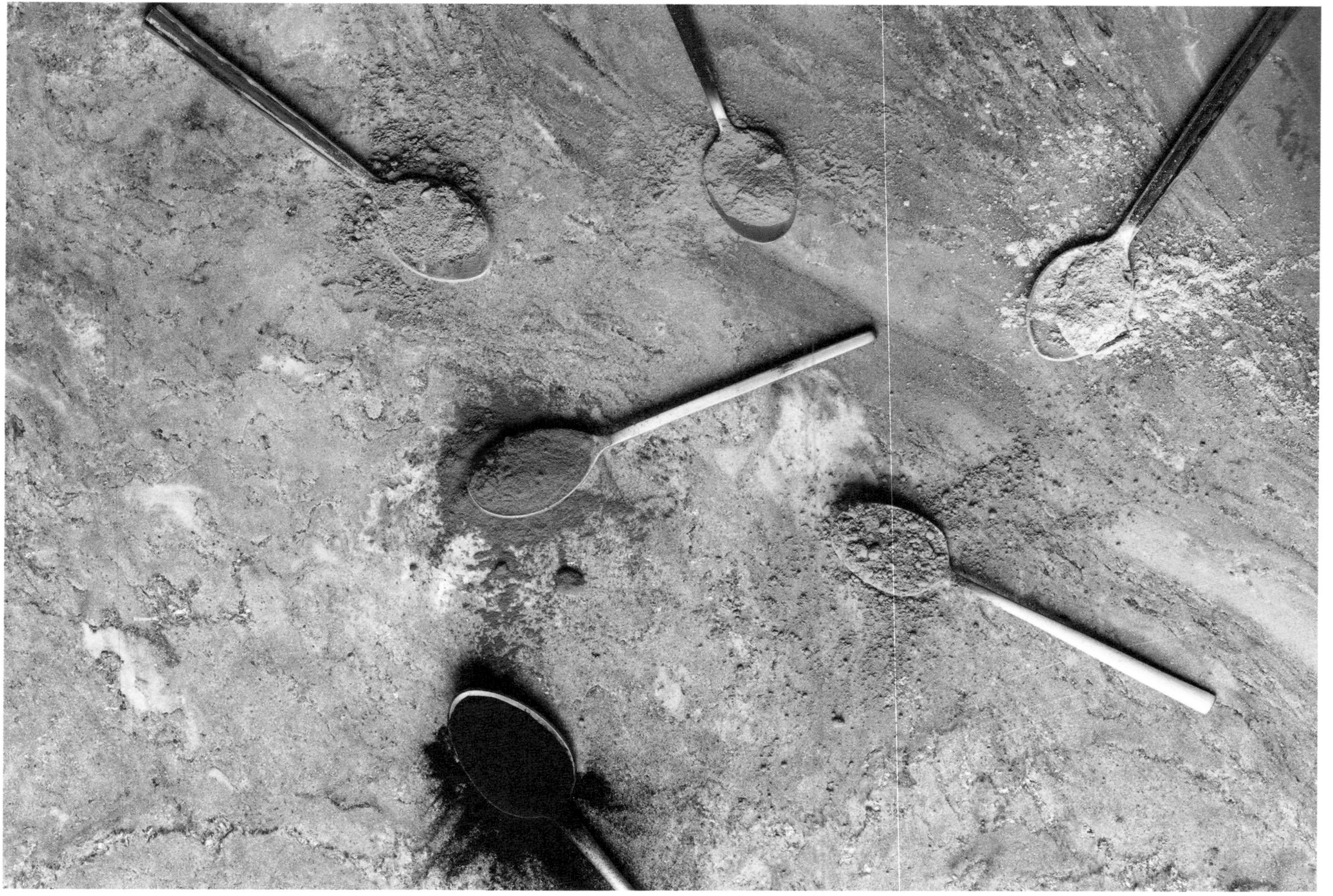

SUPERFOODS

'Superfood' is the name given to nutrient-dense foods that contain lots of vitamins, minerals and antioxidants. Although they don't cancel out an unhealthy diet they can add an extra health boost. I am a huge advocate of superfoods and think they are a great addition to any diet.

In recent years the industry has upped the prices of many superfood supplements and powders, which are now a multi-billion-pound industry, so it can be expensive and also confusing to know which superfoods are worth the money. You may find you are already eating superfoods, in everyday ingredients such as fresh fruit.

I eat the sort of everyday superfoods that can be found in any shop all the time, but I also love to use some of the more unusual ones, too. Discovering new superfoods can be fun because you have to experiment with which ingredients they work well with, as they all have different flavours. Some have a caramel taste, while others don't taste so great and need to be disguised in a fruity smoothie. It's true that superfoods have built a reputation in the media and now have the price tag to show for it, but it's all about trying different ones and seeing if they work well for you.

They don't necessarily have to be these expensive powders from health food shops; you may find you are already eating them

EVERYDAY SUPERFOODS

Blueberries	High in fibre, vitamin C and K, blueberries contain a high amount of antioxidants. Antioxidants have been shown to help to accelerate muscle recovery and reduce inflammation, making them a great post-workout snack. I add a handful to porridge, granola or smoothies.
Kale	A very nutritious and versatile food, kale is high in fibre, vitamin A, C and K, and provides a wealth of benefits including healthy skin and strengthened immune system.
Sweet Potato	These are more nutrient-dense than white potatoes, but also taste better and have a lower Glycaemic Index, meaning blood sugar levels will increase more gradually.
Garlic	For centuries, garlic has been used as a natural remedy all around the world because it acts as a natural antibiotic, fighting off viral and bacterial infections, and contains strong immune-boosting properties that help to fight off cold and flu symptoms.
Nuts	I include a lot of nuts in my recipes, because they are packed with protein, fibre and essential fats. You can eat a handful-sized portion as a snack, or you can sprinkle them over salads for texture. I have a few favourites, each with their own health benefits.
Walnuts	Notorious as one of the most super of all superfood nuts because they contain high levels of antioxidants, and healthy fats which help keep your heart, skin and hair healthy.
Almonds	Almonds are a good source of healthy fats which help to keep cholesterol levels healthy. They are also high in vitamin E and magnesium. They're great for those who avoid dairy as they are rich in calcium, which is great for bone density.

Brazil Nuts

These are so beneficial that some people actually eat 1 or 2 a day as you would a normal vitamin. They contain more selenium than another other food, a mineral high in antioxidants that may help brain function, promotes a healthy thyroid and helps keep our hair and nails healthy.

EXOTIC SUPERFOODS

Chia Seeds

Packed with fibre and protein, omega-3s and healthy fats vital for brain health. Mixed with water they swell and can be used as an egg replacer, I love to add them to smoothies, too.

Flaxseeds (Linseeds)

Another great egg replacer in baking, but use the milled version not whole seeds for a more discrete flavour and texture. High in protein, fibre, omega-3s and minerals and vitamins such as magnesium and iron.

Baobab Powder

Milled from fruit grown in Africa on the baobab tree, it's incredibly high in antioxidants, nutrients and minerals with a sherbet citrus taste. Rich in vitamin C, it provides a natural energy boost, so add a tablespoon to smoothies.

Maca Powder

Known for centuries to be a natural aphrodisiac, maca is believed to boost energy levels, balance hormones and improve moods, making it a great addition for anyone who suffers from depression, anxiety or mood disorders.

Raw Cacao Powder and Nibs

Cacao is raw, unprocessed chocolate from the cacao bean and it contains high levels of antioxidants. Do not confuse it with cocoa, which is processed and less nutritious. Research shows that cacoa helps improve circulation, cardiovascular health and mood and contains magnesium, calcium, zinc and iron.

Matcha	This powdered green tea has been used for thousands of years in Japan. Matcha is believed to speed up metabolism, is packed full with antioxidants and gives you an energy boost – a great coffee replacer.
Spirulina Powder	An excellent source of protein which helps to build and strengthen muscles, spirulina has all the essential amino acids. This algae contains powerful antioxidants and is rich in vitamins and vital minerals, particularly B vitamins.
Açaí Powder	A great superfood, açaí has a delicious berry taste and is rich in antioxidants. I love to use this in smoothies because it provides an instant hit of energy as well as vital minerals and vitamins.

HERBS

Basil	I use basil mainly in Italian recipes, including it blended up to make pesto, or in salads, and to garnish pasta dishes. It is also believed to ease stomach problems.
Coriander	This herb goes especially well with spicy Mexican and Indian dishes. It can be used fresh or you can use the powder from the seeds which can either be bought or ground at home. Both have a distinct flavour with the bonus of containing many vitamins, including vitamins A, C and K.
Mint	A very versatile herb that goes well in many sweet dishes or salads as well as in refreshing, summery drinks. Mint has been used for thousands of years for its medicinal properties, notably soothing stomach aches and pains.

Parsley

This is a herb with delicate flavours that I find works well in fresh salads. It is rich in vital vitamins, antioxidants and minerals that help reduce the risk of diseases.

Rosemary

I love to roast vegetables in fresh rosemary. The smell it creates always reminds me of Christmas! Besides being one of the most flavoursome herbs, it is also known for boosting memory and mood.

Thyme

This is one of those herbs that seems to go with everything, but I particularly like pairing it with bananas in sweet recipes, such as my flapjacks (see page 221). The essential oils in thyme have also been connected to helping cure bacterial infections.

Oregano

I use this herb in its dried form for lots of recipes; try my Squashetti + 'Meatballs' (see page 104) and Mexican Chilli Bowl, (see page 99).

Mixed Herbs

You can get packets of dried mixed herbs easily in the supermarket. These are great to have on hand in your store cupboard to add a hit of flavour to any dish.

SPICES

Cayenne Pepper	I use the dried, ground version of this hot red chilli pepper to add a hit of spiciness. Cayenne is rich in antioxidants and is believed to improve circulation.
Chilli Powder	Simply dried and ground chillies – a quick, easy way to spice up your meals when you don't have any fresh chillies.
Cinnamon	I use ground cinnamon in many of my recipes, mainly because I love the taste, but also because it is rich in antioxidants and is believed to improve metabolism and reduce inflammation.
Cumin	I use ground cumin or whole seeds in many recipes for its nutty, earthy taste. Its essential oils also help promote healthy digestion.
Ginger	I use ground ginger where I don't want the bulkiness and moisture of fresh ginger but still want the flavour.
Paprika	There are many types available, ranging from sweet to smoky and spicy. I choose regular or smoked paprika rather than hot; if I fancy some heat I'll add a pinch of cayenne pepper. Paprika is high in vitamin C, which helps keep skin healthy.
Turmeric	This adds a vibrant yellow colour to dishes. It has been used for hundreds of years for its medicinal properties, notably its anti-inflammatory effects – I've even cured an infected finger by adding turmeric to it and wrapping it in cloth and then cling film overnight!
Pure Vanilla Extract or Powder	A great addition to any sweet recipe, particularly cakes and biscuits. Nothing beats the flavour of the seeds straight from the pod, but these can be expensive. I usually use powder, ground beans or pure extract.

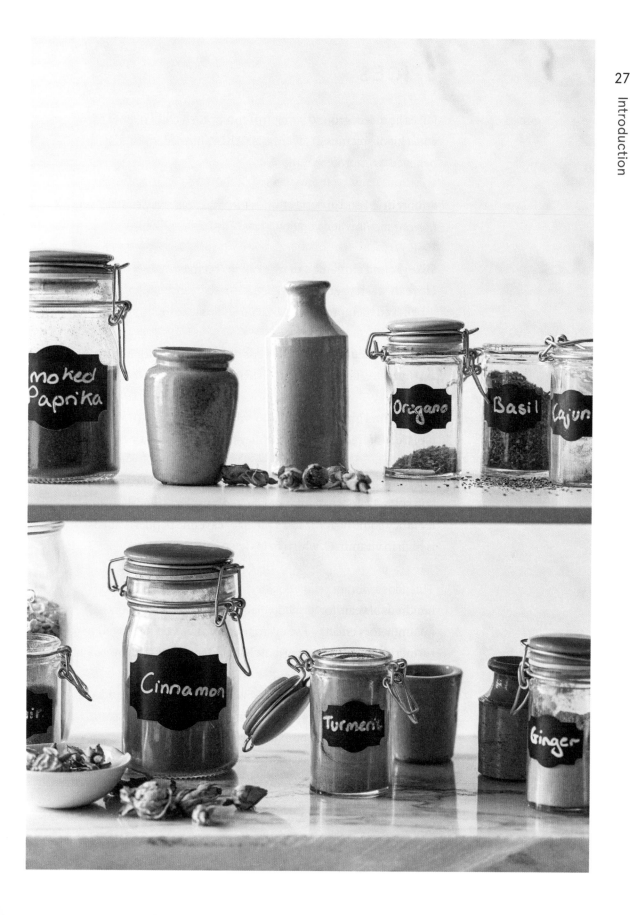
Paprika
Oregano
Basil
Cinnamon
Ginger

STAPLES

One of the biggest barriers people find to changing the way they eat is the myth that healthy recipes need expensive, obscure ingredients. While eating healthily can be expensive if you're constantly buying the superfood of the moment, it doesn't have to break the bank. Once you stock up with staple ingredients that'll keep for a long time in your cupboards, you'll only need to buy fruit and vegetables fresh. When I changed the way I ate I noticed how much money I was saving by not buying meat, seafood and dairy.

Most of my recipes are made with fresh, wholesome ingredients that can be found in your local supermarket

I bought most of the ingredients in this book from the little supermarket near me. So don't worry about needing to hunt these down – most supermarkets have a healthy or 'free-from' aisle containing everything from quinoa and bulgar wheat to dairy-free milks and yoghurts. I do like to go to health food shops occasionally, though, because the quality can be better and they have my favourite brands.

There will be some ingredients here that you might not have cooked with before, such as black rice, but these are easy to find and surprisingly simple to cook. Once you've tried them a few times, I guarantee these will become favourite staples.

Occasionally I use ingredients such as coconut sugar that are harder to find in smaller supermarkets. So rather than traipsing around shops trying to find these, order them online to find the best deal and perhaps buy in bulk to save money, too. Here are a few shops that I buy my ingredients from, some of which you can shop from online: Whole Foods Market, Planet Organic, Holland & Barrett, Amazon, buywholefoodsonline.co.uk.

FOOD CUPBOARD STAPLES

I use whole black peppercorns in a grinder.	Black Pepper
This is less processed and refined than table salt. It is also higher in many minerals such as boron, zinc and phosphorus needed for healthy hair, nails, skin and thyroid function. I always taste my dishes before seasoning and try to use as little salt as possible.	Pink Himalayan Salt
This is natural, unrefined and contains many essential mineral elements. If you don't have pink Himalayan salt, use this instead.	Sea Salt
This oil is highly resistant to oxidation at high heat levels so it is ideal for cooking with. It has been claimed coconut oil has remarkable health benefits and I find it's lovely to cook with because it adds a lovely subtle flavour to all kinds of dishes.	Raw Unrefined Coconut Oil
Delicious as a dressing on salads or raw pestos. I tend to cook with coconut oil and use extra-virgin olive oil in cold, raw dishes.	Extra-virgin Olive Oil
This is my non-dairy milk of choice; I love the taste, it goes well with porridge or cereal and helps thicken dishes. Rice milk and coconut milk are delicious alternatives.	Unsweetened Almond Milk
I buy natural and organic almond butter without added sugar or salt and use it in desserts or cookies, in smoothies for a protein kick or on crackers as an afternoon snack.	Almond Butter
I always make sure I am well stocked with oats. I buy rolled, gluten-free oats. I also grind them into a flour and bake with it.	Oats
My grain of choice; it is so versatile and a complete protein. I use it instead of white rice or pasta, cold and mixed into salads or in stews. I've also made a granola with it (see page 46).	Quinoa
I use the tinned version and always full-fat so that it's as close to its natural form as possible. It's brilliant for adding creaminess to soups, curries and desserts.	Coconut Milk

Maple Syrup	This is a 100% natural and pure sweetener straight from the maple tree, retaining many of its minerals and antioxidants. It has a lovely, distinctive flavour that adds depth to baked goods. Try to use pure versions rather than maple-flavoured syrups.
Coconut Sugar (or Palm Sugar)	A great 100% less refined replacement for white sugar. Although more expensive, a little goes a long way, so it lasts longer. It offers more nutrients and minerals and has a lower Glycaemic Index.
Buckwheat Flour	I avoid using plain flour because it's so heavily processed and contains few nutritional benefits. Buckwheat flour can be used for pancakes, muffins and many other baked goods.
Spelt Flour	A great alternative to plain flour; it contains many more nutrients and is high in protein and fibre.
Dates	With their delicious caramel flavour, many minerals and vitamins and high fibre content, dates are so versatile. I buy Medjool dates because they tend to be plump and moist.
Nuts	Almonds and cashews are my favourites because they contain a high level of protein and nutrients. The raw, unsalted versions without oil are the most nutritious.
Brown Rice	This type of rice is slower to digest then white rice, releasing energy slowly; it is also higher in fibre and protein.
Apple Cider Vinegar	This tastes especially good in salad dressings. It has many health benefits and it is believed to significantly help digestion. Surprisingly, it's also good as a raising agent in baking as it reacts with baking powder.
Nutritional Yeast	Ignore the off-putting name, this is a great source of vitamin B12. It has a cheesy flavour that can be used as a Parmesan replacer. Get the version that says it's fortified with B12. It's also high in fibre, protein, is gluten-free and contains folic acid.

FRESH STAPLES

Research shows that garlic has many health benefits including anti-inflammatory, antiviral and antibacterial properties. For me, nothing beats a strong garlic kick, so I add it to many of my recipes.	Garlic
I use fresh ginger a lot. It contains many minerals and vitamins and has been used for millennia to calm stomach issues.	Ginger
These citrus fruits have amazing antioxidant properties. Add them to juices, salads or even curries to reap their health benefits.	Lemons and Limes
I always have these around to add to my pre-workout morning smoothies for sweetness and to create a thick, creamy texture. This potassium-rich fruit is higher in carbs, making you feel fuller for longer, slowly releasing energy into the body. I wait until they are ripe with brown spots before I use them, and if they get over-ripe, I freeze them, peeled and cut into chunks, to use another time, usually in my Açaí Bowl (see page 37).	Bananas
These are always in my fridge. I love the taste and they are also very high in antioxidants, so I scatter them over my porridge or granola .	Blueberries
Less starchy than white potatoes, these are delicious and richer in nutrients. They also taste incredibly good, so I eat them about three times a week, sometimes more!	Sweet Potatoes
Rich in many vitamins and minerals, particularly iron. A great way to make the most of this is to add a handful of raw leaves to a smoothie exploiting their mild taste.	Spinach
Of course, this classic 'superfood' vegetable is one of my staples. I like to add this to smoothies and juices for an added health kick. I also like to steam it as a side dish at dinner or eat it for lunch with a squeeze of fresh lemon.	Kale

CORE EQUIPMENT

Blender	A NutriBullet is a great addition to any kitchen. I use it to make my smoothies and also use the milling blade to make pesto, crush nuts and grind oats into flour.
Juicer	For smooth juices, use a juicer that extracts the pulp. Prices vary hugely, but they start from £20.
Food Processor	Not an absolute necessity, but the more you get into cooking the more you may find this makes life a lot easier. I love my food processor for making anything from cake batters and burger mixtures to creamy cashew cheese and pestos. Again, prices vary, but you can get cheap ones that do a good job.
Spiralizer	I'm a big fan of spiralizing vegetables – where vegetables are turned into long noodle-like shapes as a great alternative to pasta or to make salads more exciting. You can buy these quite cheaply for about £15.
Measuring Cups	This is probably the most used and loved piece of equipment in my kitchen. I use measuring cups instead of scales as I find them quicker and more convenient. Although not traditionally a British way of measuring, you can find them in most department stores and kitchen stores for under £5.
Measuring Spoons	I like the ease and precision of using these, but you can also just use your usual teaspoons and tablespoons, as long as you keep consistent while cooking.
Garlic Mincer	I find this so useful because it takes a fraction of the amount of time of hand-chopping but also prevents you getting that strong garlic smell on your fingers. You can find these in most kitchen shops.
Vegetable Peeler	A pretty obvious one, but a staple in my kitchen nonetheless.

If you don't want to fork out for a food processor, I would recommend purchasing a pestle and mortar to crush nuts and seeds.	Pestle and Mortar
To get the most nutrients from your vegetables, steam rather than boil. You can buy electric steamers, but I have always used a three-tiered stainless-steel steamer that you place on the hob, which are a fraction of the price.	Steamer
It is important to get some good-quality non-stick pans. Although slightly more expensive, they last longer, therefore justifying the price in my opinion.	Non-stick Pans
I have 2 basic baking trays and 2 roasting trays which range in size from 35–39cm.	Roasting and Baking Trays
I use 20cm diameter, springform cake tins – so you can unclip the sides and they also have a loose bottom so you can release the cake easily. I also have a few baking tins ranging in size from 20-25cm.	Baking Tin
I have a couple of different-sized loaf tins, but usually I use a 18 x 8cm one.	Loaf Tin
I use a 22cm enamel pie dish.	Pie Dish

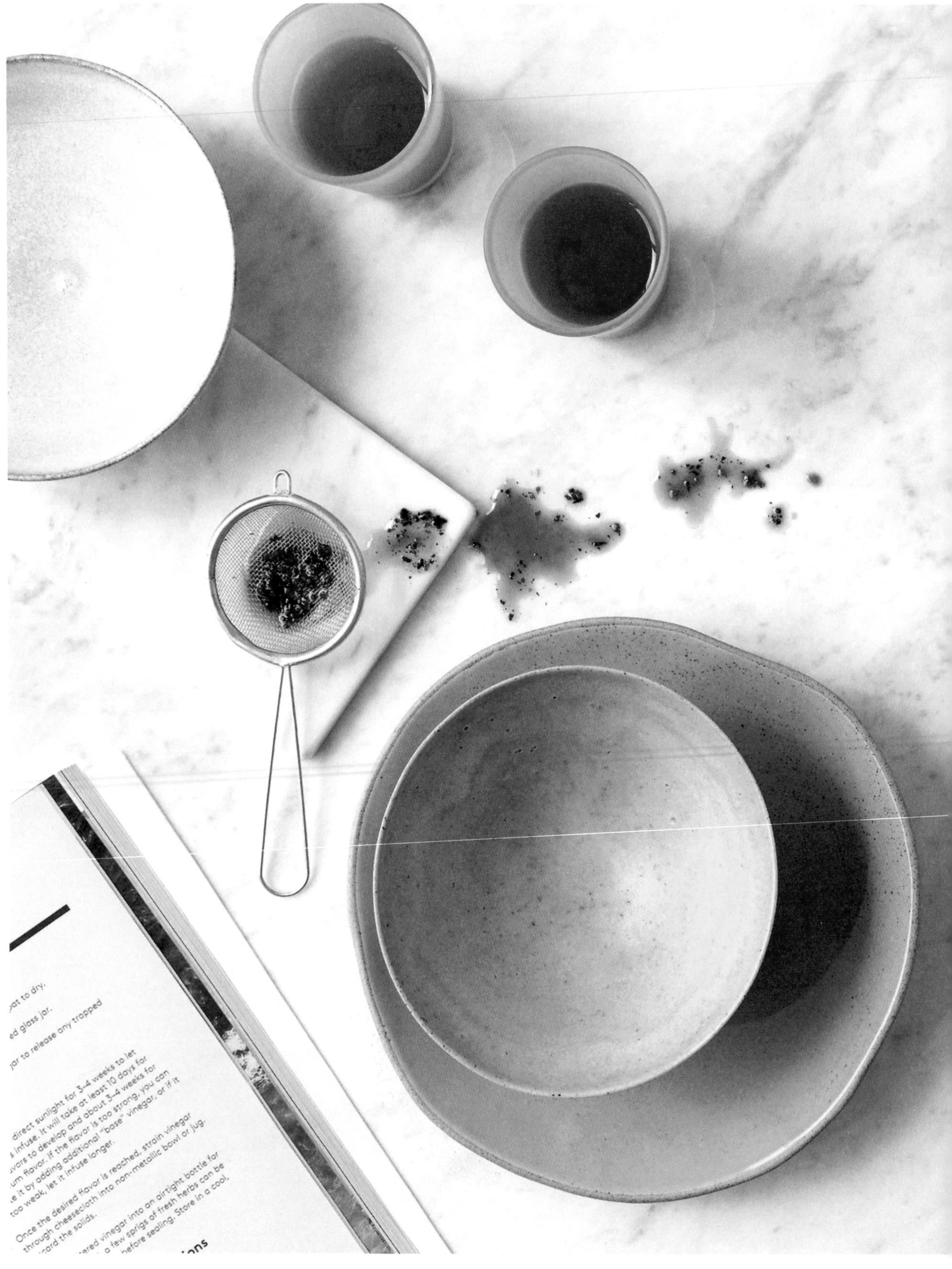
to dry.
glass jar.
to release any trapped
direct sunlight for 3–4 weeks to let
infuse. It will take at least 10 days for
to develop and about 3–4 weeks for
flavor. If the flavor is too strong, you can
it by adding additional "base" vinegar, or if it
too weak, let it infuse longer.
Once the desired flavor is reached, strain vinegar
through cheesecloth into non-metallic bowl or jug.
the solids.
vinegar into an airtight bottle for
a few sprigs of fresh herbs can be
sealing. Store in a cool,

Breakfast

01

SMOOTHIE BOWLS – 3 WAYS

I first discovered smoothie bowls in LA at a quirky cafe called Juice Generation and the best I've ever tasted were in Bali. They were a revelation to me and since then I've made my own versions, trying out different combinations of fruit and superfoods.

AÇAÍ

Serves 2

Ingredients

3 frozen bananas, peeled
50g (¼ cup) fresh or frozen blueberries, raspberries and blackberries
125ml (½ cup) unsweetened almond milk
2 tbsp açaí powder
2 tbsp maca powder (optional)

SUPERFOOD CHOCOLATE

Serves 2

Ingredients

3 frozen bananas, peeled, chopped
1 tbsp raw cacao powder
1 tbsp chia seeds
1 tbsp lucuma powder (optional)
125ml (½ cup) unsweetened almond milk

TROPICAL

Serves 2

Ingredients

a large handful of spinach
100g (½ cup) frozen mango chunks
100g (½ cup) frozen pineapple chunks
¼ cucumber
60ml (¼ cup) coconut water, plus extra if needed
2 ice cubes
1 tsp baobab powder (optional)
1 tsp spirulina (optional)

1. Simply place all the ingredients in a blender (make sure your blender can work with frozen fruit).
2. Whizz until creamy and smooth, adding extra almond milk or coconut water, if needed.
3. Serve in bowls, decorated with toppings of your choice.

Tip ... When bananas get over-ripe, peel and roughly chop them, place in a freezer bag and freeze so you have them to make smoothie bowls.

Topping ideas ...
Sliced banana
Fresh berries
Dried mulberries
Goji berries
Sunflower seeds
Pumpkin seeds
Chia seeds
Hemp seeds
Coconut flakes
Almond butter
Homemade granola (see page 46)

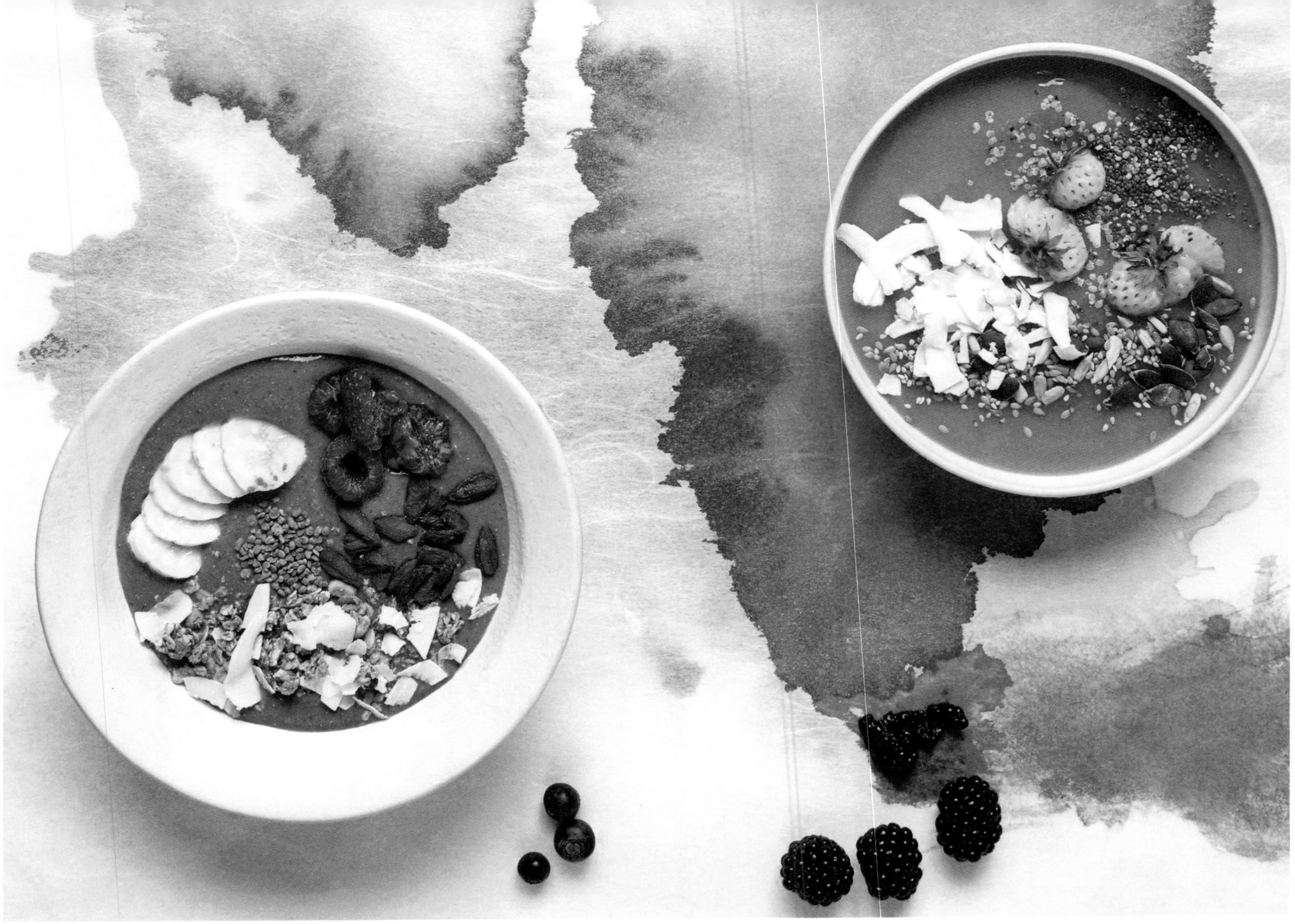

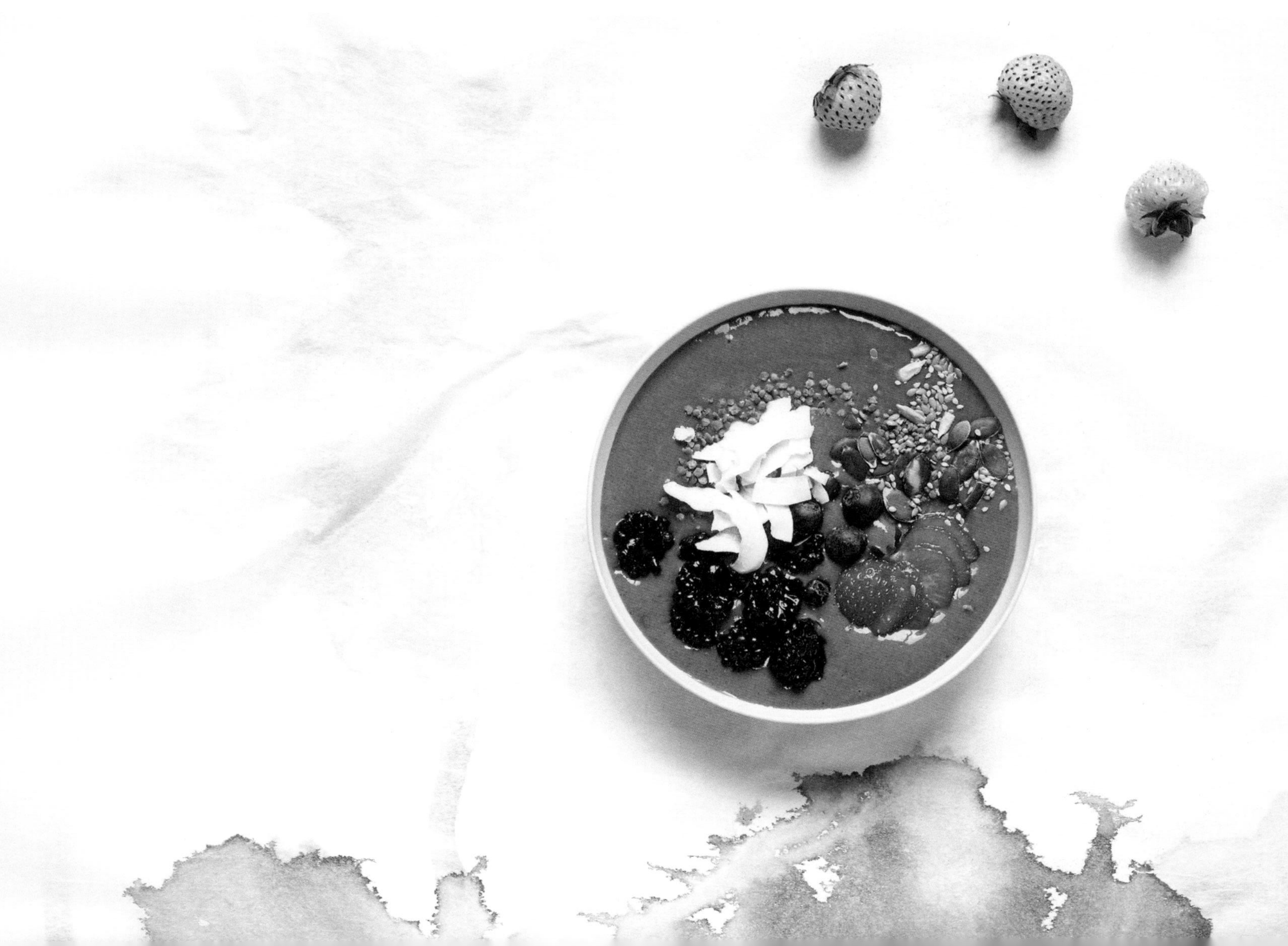

PORRIDGE – 3 WAYS

I'm a huge fan of porridge – it's one of the best breakfasts, providing so much energy that it usually keeps me going until lunch. I like experimenting with different flavours. Inspired by traditional British puddings, because who doesn't want to eat dessert for breakfast when it's good for you?

BANANA BREAD

Serves 2

Ingredients

100g (1 cup) rolled oats
250ml (1 cup) unsweetened almond milk
1 ripe banana, peeled
30g (¼ cup) raisins
1 tsp ground cinnamon
¼ tsp ground nutmeg
1 tsp maca powder (optional)

1. Place the oats, almond milk and 250ml (1 cup) water into a small saucepan and place over a medium-low heat.
2. Thinly slice and stir in half the banana with the raisins, cinnamon, nutmeg and maca powder, if using. Cook for 5-7 minutes, or until thick and creamy and the oats have absorbed all the liquid, stirring regularly.
3. Thinly slice the remaining banana and serve the porridge topped with the banana slices and any other toppings you like.

Serving ideas ...
A teaspoon of my homemade Strawberry Chia Jam (see page 56).

CARROT CAKE

Serves 2

Ingredients

100g (1 cup) rolled oats
250ml (1 cup) unsweetened almond milk
1 carrot, peeled and grated
1 tbsp date syrup or maple syrup
¼ tsp each of ground cinnamon, ground nutmeg and ground ginger
30g (¼ cup) raisins

1. Put the oats, almond milk and 250ml (1 cup) water into a small saucepan and place over a medium heat.
2. Stir in most of the carrot along with the syrup, cinnamon, nutmeg, ginger and raisins. Cook for 5–7 minutes, or until thick and creamy, stirring regularly.
3. Serve sprinkled with the remaining carrot and any other toppings that you like.

Serving ideas ...
A small handful of chopped unsalted raw walnuts.

CHERRY BAKEWELL

Serves 2

Ingredients

100g (1 cup) rolled oats
250ml (1 cup) unsweetened almond milk
4 fresh cherries, stoned
1 tbsp almond butter
1 tbsp ground almonds
1 tsp organic vanilla extract
1 tbsp maple syrup

Serving ideas ...
A small handful of chopped almonds.
Fresh cherries, stoned and halved.

1. Put the oats, almond milk and 250ml (1 cup) water into a small saucepan and set over a medium heat.
2. Roughly chop the cherries and stir into the saucepan with the almond butter, ground almonds, vanilla extract and maple syrup. Cook for 5–6 minutes, or until thick and creamy, stirring regularly.

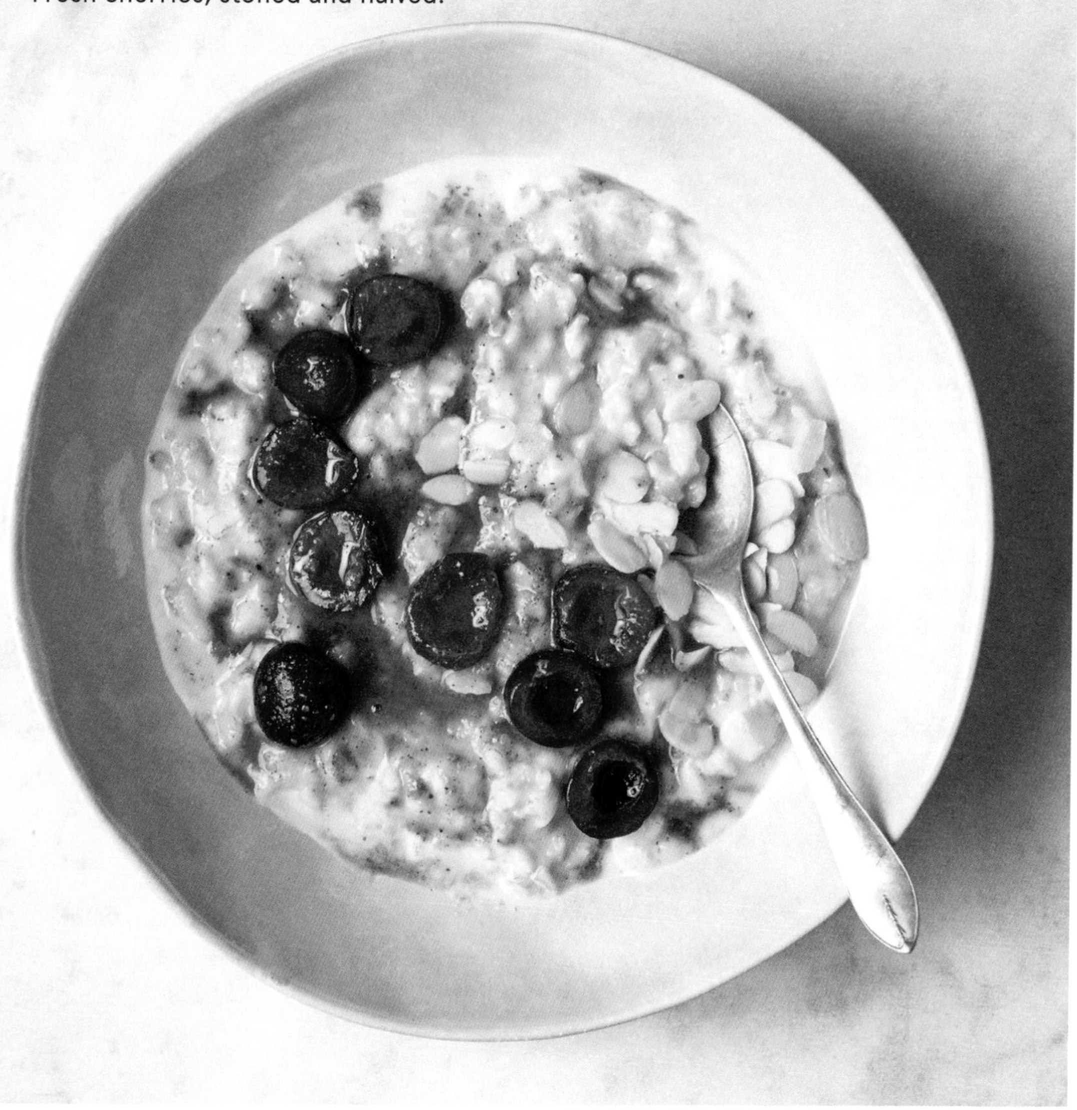

SMOOTH BANANA + BLUEBERRY OATMEAL

Serves 2

Oatmeal can be used to describe oat porridge as we know it, but can also mean a smoother consistency, using ground oats. I love this banana-flavoured oatmeal, which is easily made by blending all the ingredients until smooth. The whole blueberries, once heated, burst and provide a delicious pop of flavour.

Ingredients

2 ripe bananas, peeled
100g (1 cup) rolled oats
500ml (2 cups) unsweetened almond milk
1 tsp ground cinnamon
150g (1 cup) blueberries

1. In a blender, whizz 1½ bananas with the oats, almond milk and cinnamon until smooth.
2. Pour into a small saucepan and stir in the blueberries.
3. Set the saucepan over a low heat and cook for 5–6 minutes, or until thick and creamy, stirring regularly.
4. Slice the remaining half of the banana and serve on top of the oatmeal with your preferred topping.

Topping ideas ...
Almond butter
Fresh blueberries
Pumpkin seeds

PEAR QUINOA PORRIDGE

Serves 2

Quinoa is now widely known as a superfood grain. It's a complete protein, which means it contains all the nine amino acids that we need, which is rare for a plant-based food. I wanted to use it to create a breakfast, and as I'm a porridge fanatic, I came up with this warming, subtly sweet dish, served with pear for a lovely fresh taste.

Ingredients

100g (½ cup) quinoa, rinsed
375ml (1½ cups) unsweetened almond milk, plus extra (optional)
2 ripe pears, cored
juice of ½ lemon
1 tsp ground cinnamon
1 tsp vanilla powder or 2 tsp organic vanilla extract
a handful of chopped unsalted raw walnuts, to serve
maple syrup (optional), to serve

1. Tip the quinoa into a saucepan with the almond milk and 125ml (½ cup) water and place over a medium-high heat. Bring to the boil, then turn the heat down to low and simmer for 15 minutes, stirring occasionally, until the liquid has been absorbed and the quinoa is cooked, adding extra almond milk if needed.
2. Thinly slice a quarter of one of the pears and keep to one side. Chop the rest of the pear and the remaining pear into small chunks and stir into the cooked porridge with the lemon juice, cinnamon and vanilla.
3. Serve sprinkled with the chopped walnuts and the sliced pear. Drizzle with maple syrup if you fancy something sweeter.

Tip ... To help reduce the earthy taste quinoa sometimes has, simply tip the rinsed quinoa into a dry pan over a low heat and gently fry off the moisture for a few seconds, shaking often and being careful to not let the quinoa burn.

OVERNIGHT OAT POTS – 3 WAYS

If you often find yourself skipping breakfast in the mornings, why not make an overnight breakfast jar? I throw these together in the evening and overnight the oats plump up and the flavours intensify. In the morning I can grab and go!

APPLE + BLUEBERRY

Serves 1

Ingredients

creamy oat layer

½ apple, cored and grated
50g (½ cup) rolled oats
125ml (½ cup) unsweetened almond milk
½ tsp ground cinnamon

blueberry layer

1 tbsp chia seeds
80g (½ cup) blueberries
2cm piece of fresh ginger, peeled and finely grated
2 tsp açaí powder (optional)
a handful of blueberries, to serve
a handful of chopped unsalted raw macadamia nuts, to serve

1. Mix together the apple, oats, almond milk and cinnamon and set aside.
2. Mix the chia seeds with 5 tablespoons of water in a bowl. Mash the blueberries with a fork and add to the chia with the ginger and açaí powder, if using.
3. Spoon half the oat mixture into a large 500ml jar or glass and layer up with half the blueberry mixture. Repeat until used up.
4. Seal with a lid or cover and keep in the fridge overnight. By the morning it'll be ready to eat. Sprinkle over the toppings and dig in.

STRAWBERRIES + 'CREAM'

Serves 1

Ingredients

strawberry layer

6 strawberries, stalks removed

creamy oat layer

½ ripe banana, peeled
50g (½ cup) rolled oats
125ml (½ cup) unsweetened almond milk
¼ x 400g tin coconut milk
¼ tsp vanilla powder or ½ tsp organic vanilla extract

1. Thinly slice the strawberries and mash the banana with the back of a fork.
2. Mix the mashed banana in a bowl with the remaining ingredients apart from the strawberries.
3. Spoon a third of the creamy oat mixture into a large 500ml jar or glass. Layer with a few of the strawberries and add another layer of the oat mixture. Repeat until used up.
4. Seal with a lid or cover and keep in the fridge overnight. By morning the oats will have thickened up ready for you to dig in.

Tip ... Freeze the leftover banana half for a smoothie bowl another time.

PINK BERRY

Serves 1

Ingredients

125g (1 cup) raspberries
1 heaped tsp açaí powder (optional)
250ml (1 cup) unsweetened almond milk
50g (½ cup) rolled oats
3 tbsp chia seeds
1 tbsp goji berries
a small handful of unsalted raw pistachios, to serve

1. In a blender or NutriBullet, whizz the fresh berries, açaí powder, if using, and almond milk until smooth.
2. Pour into a large 500ml jar or glass and stir in the oats, chia seeds and goji berries. Seal with the lid and keep in the fridge overnight.
3. In the morning, sprinkle with the pistachios and dig in.

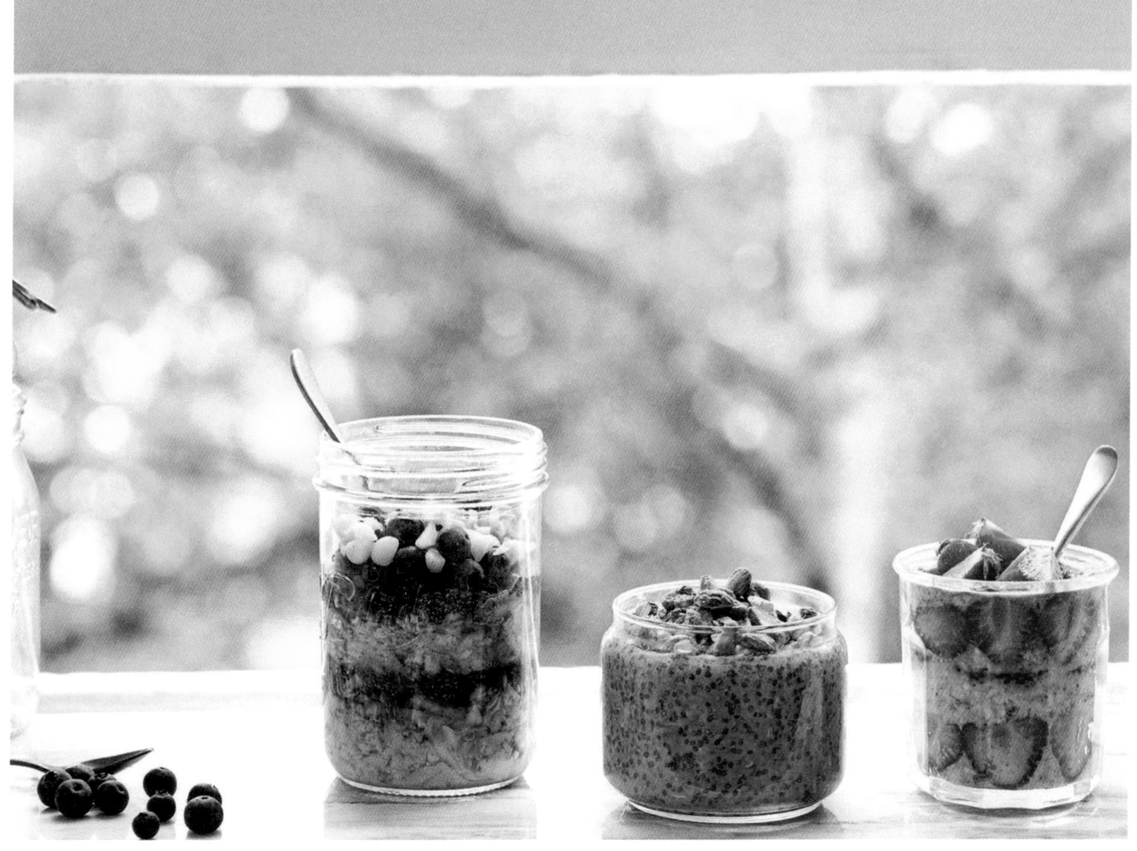

GRANOLA

I make this at the weekend and store it in an airtight container – ready to go at all times. It will last a few weeks but it's so moreish it's usually gone before that! My cacao and coconut version of granola makes me feel like a kid with chocolaty cereal. And yes, you get the same choco milk effect!

CACAO + COCONUT

Makes 16 servings

Ingredients

4 tbsp coconut oil
4 tbsp maple syrup
4 tbsp unsweetened almond milk
30g (¼ cup) raw cacao powder
300g (3 cups) rolled oats
30g (½ cup) coconut flakes
100g (½ cup) quinoa, rinsed
25g (¼ cup) desiccated coconut
30g (¼ cup) raw cacao nibs

1. Preheat the oven to 170°C/325°F/gas 3.
2. Heat the coconut oil in a small saucepan over a low heat until melted, then stir in the maple syrup, almond milk and cacao powder and remove from the heat.
3. Stir together the oats, coconut flakes, quinoa, desiccated coconut and cacao nibs. Pour the wet mixture into the bowl and stir until everything is fully coated.
4. Pour into a baking tray and gently press the mixture down with the back of a wooden spoon.
5. Bake in the hot oven for 30 minutes, stirring occasionally, then remove from the oven and allow to cool.

MIXED FRUIT + NUT

Makes 16 servings

Ingredients

4 tbsp coconut oil
125ml (½ cup) maple syrup
200g (2 cups) rolled oats
160g (1 cup) unsalted raw almonds
100g (1 cup) unsalted raw pecan nuts
60g (½ cup) pumpkin seeds
30g (½ cup) coconut flakes
120g (1 cup) chopped dried fruit, such as unsulphured apricots, medjool dates, figs, raisins and prunes

1. Preheat the oven to 170°C/325°F/gas 3.
2. Heat the coconut oil in a small saucepan over a low heat until melted, then stir in the maple syrup and remove from the heat.
3. Stir together the oats, almonds, pecan nuts and pumpkin seeds.
4. Pour the melted coconut oil and maple syrup mixture into the bowl and stir to fully coat. Then pour into a baking tray and press down with the back of a wooden spoon.
5. Bake in the hot oven for 30 minutes, stirring occasionally. Add the coconut flakes after 15 minutes. Remove from the oven and allow to cool. Stir in the dried fruit and store in an airtight container.

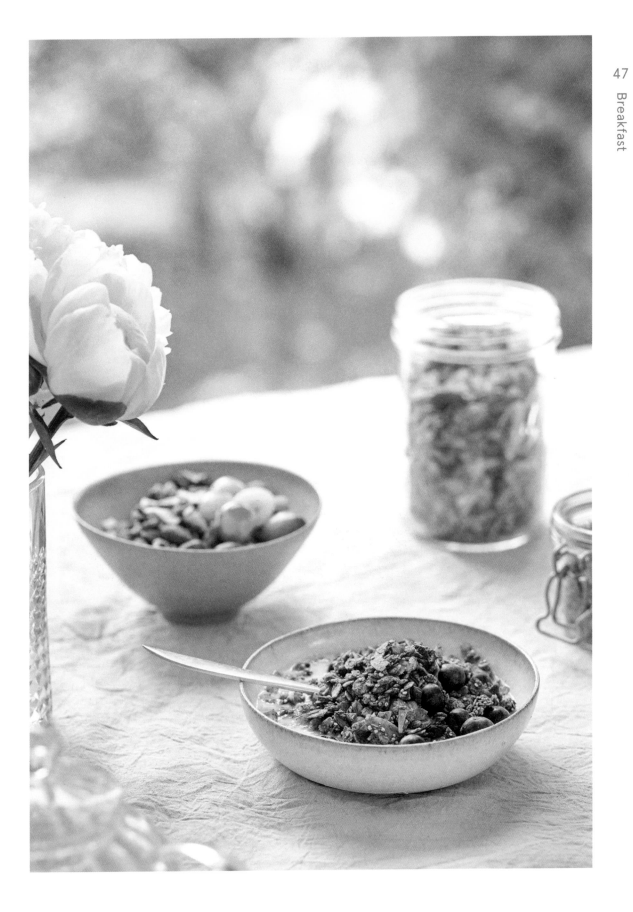

MUESLI

Makes 12 servings

As a serial cereal eater, this is my go-to breakfast during the week. Muesli is one of those things you often just buy ready made, but it's so easy to throw together. Why not make it at the weekend and set yourself up with a wholesome breakfast for the next few mornings?

Ingredients

- 100g (1 cup) rolled oats
- 30g (1 cup) puffed brown rice
- 100g (1 cup) rye flakes or barley flakes
- 50g (½ cup) flaked almonds
- 50g (½ cup) goji berries
- 30g (½ cup) coconut flakes
- 30g (¼ cup) dried cranberries or sultanas
- 30g (¼ cup) sunflower seeds
- ½ tsp ground cinnamon

1. Tip all the ingredients into a large bowl, mix together and store in an airtight container. That's it!

Serving ideas …

Almond milk and a handful of mixed fresh berries.

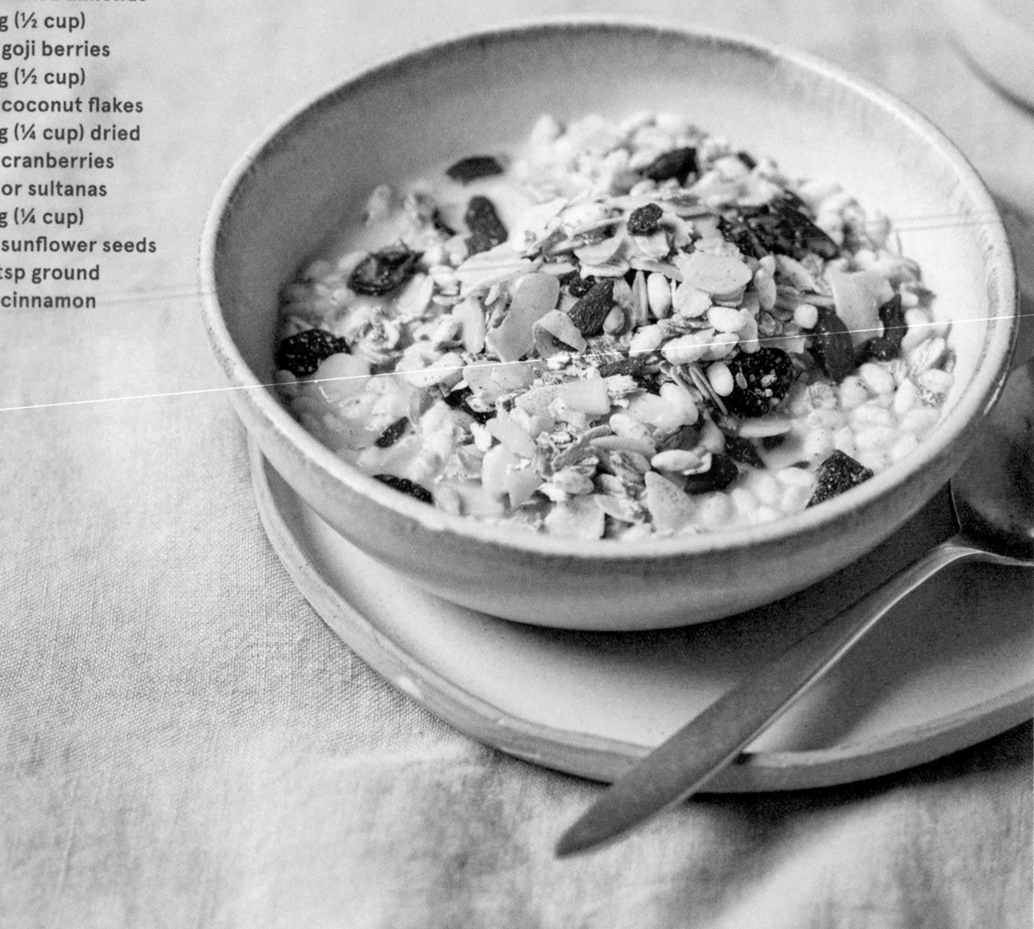

SWISS BIRCHER MUESLI

Serves 2

In the summer I crave a refreshing, light breakfast. This muesli is perfect; you only need to take it out of the fridge in the morning, grab a spoon and tuck in. My traditional Swiss recipe uses only natural sugars from the fruit and no dairy products. Try mixing it up with different toppings!

Ingredients

1 red apple
1 tbsp lemon juice
½ tsp ground cinnamon
40g (¼ cup) unsalted raw almonds
100g (1 cup) rolled oats
30g (¼ cup) raisins
1 heaped tbsp golden linseed/flaxseed
1 heaped tbsp sunflower seeds
500ml (2 cups) unsweetened almond or rice milk

1. Core the apple and grate into a large bowl, then add the lemon juice and cinnamon and mix together.
2. Crush the almonds into small chunks in a pestle and mortar or food processor. Add to the bowl with the remaining ingredients and mix well.
3. Cover with cling film and keep in the fridge overnight.
4. In the morning the oats will have soaked up the milk to become lovely and creamy. This is a perfect breakfast to take with you on-the-go. Just transfer a portion into a little jar and top with whatever you fancy.

Topping ideas ...

Pomegranate seeds
Fresh berries
Sliced banana

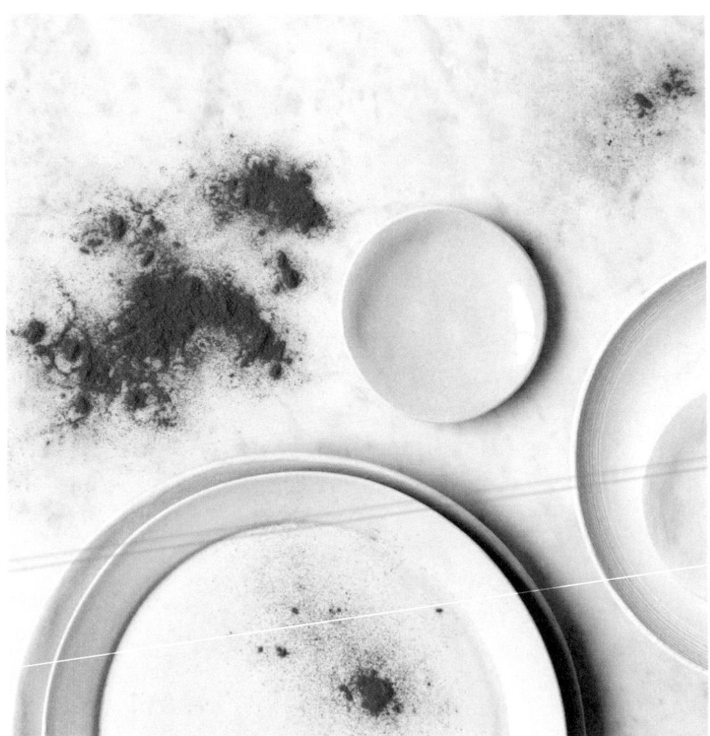

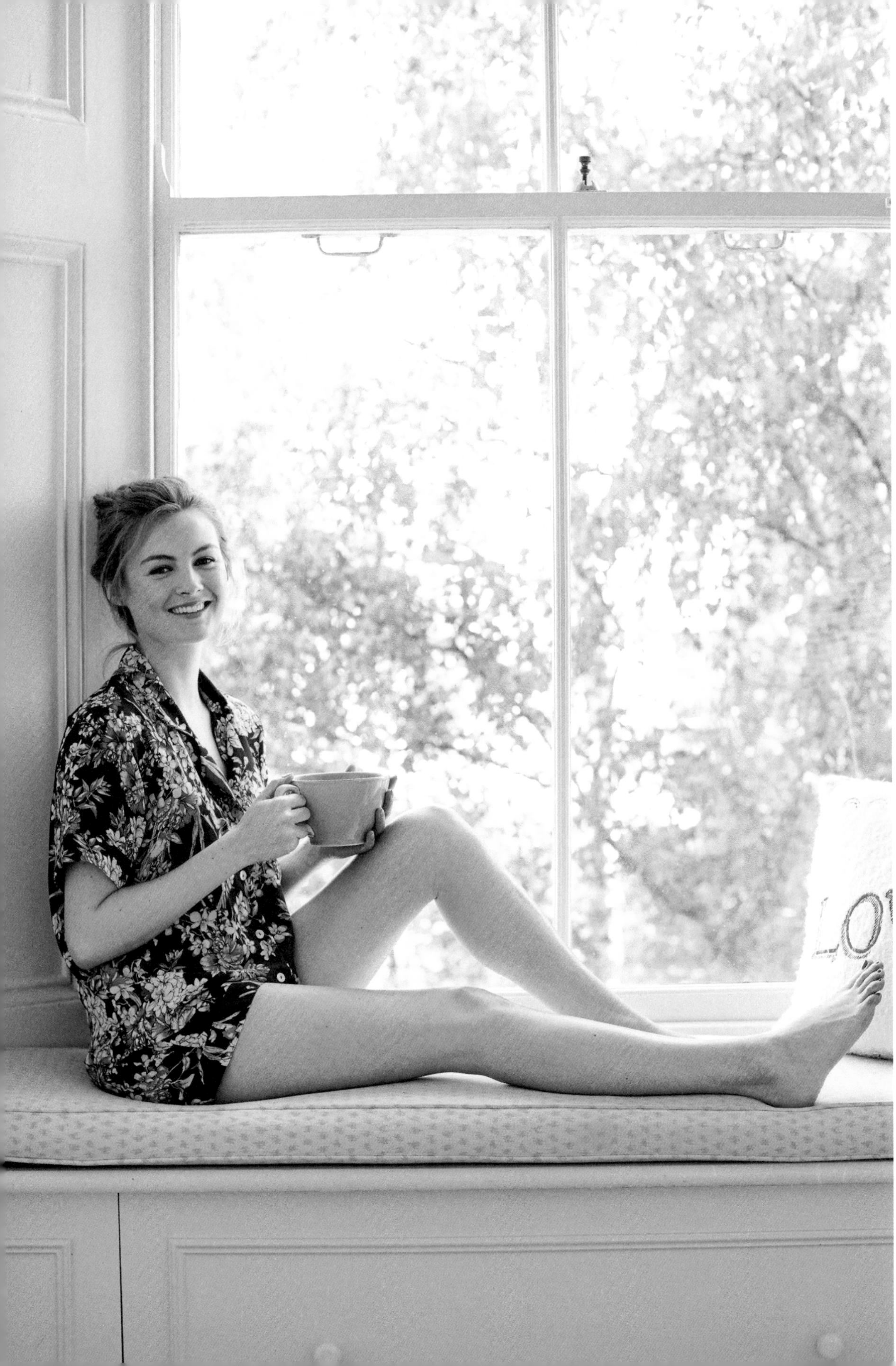

ONION + SUN-DRIED TOMATO MUFFINS

Makes 9

I love cooking savoury versions of dishes that are usually sweet. The sun-dried tomatoes, onions and herbs all work really well together to create a delicious muffin. I either make these for weekend brunch or in the evening, ready for breakfast the next day.

Ingredients

4 tbsp coconut oil, plus extra for greasing and frying
2½ tbsp milled flaxseed
½ onion, finely diced
1 garlic clove, peeled and crushed
200g (1½ cups) buckwheat flour, sifted
2 tsp baking powder
1 tbsp nutritional yeast (optional)
50g (¼ cup) sun-dried tomatoes in oil, finely chopped
25g (¼ cup) black olives, pitted and finely chopped
1 tsp each of dried rosemary, thyme and oregano
125ml (½ cup) unsweetened almond milk
150g (¾ cup) unsweetened apple sauce
2 tsp apple cider vinegar
1 tsp bicarbonate of soda
pink Himalayan salt or sea salt and freshly ground black pepper

1. Preheat the oven to 180°C/350°F/gas 4. Lightly grease nine holes of a muffin tray with coconut oil and line with muffin cases or greaseproof paper.
2. Mix the flaxseed with 4 tablespoons of water and set aside to thicken; this will act as the egg.
3. Heat a small amount of coconut oil in a frying pan, add the onion and fry for 5-7 minutes over a medium-high heat, stirring occasionally. Add the garlic and fry for a further 2 minutes, then remove from the heat.
4. In a large bowl, mix the flour with the baking powder, nutritional yeast, if using, sun-dried tomatoes, olives and herbs, add a pinch of salt and black pepper and mix well.
5. Pour the milk, coconut oil and apple sauce into a saucepan over a medium-low heat and heat gently, until the coconut oil has melted and the milk is warmed but not boiling. Remove from the heat and keep to one side.
6. In a small bowl, mix the vinegar with the bicarbonate of soda and stir until it foams; this will help the muffins rise.
7. Add the milk and apple sauce mixture to the bowl of dry ingredients, along with the vinegar and soda mixture, the flaxseed egg and the cooked onions and garlic.
8. Very gently fold to combine (this keeps the muffins nice and light – mixing too much can make them tough).
9. Divide the mixture between the muffin cases and bake in the hot oven for 25-30 minutes until a knife inserted comes out clean. Remove from the oven and place on a wire rack to cool.

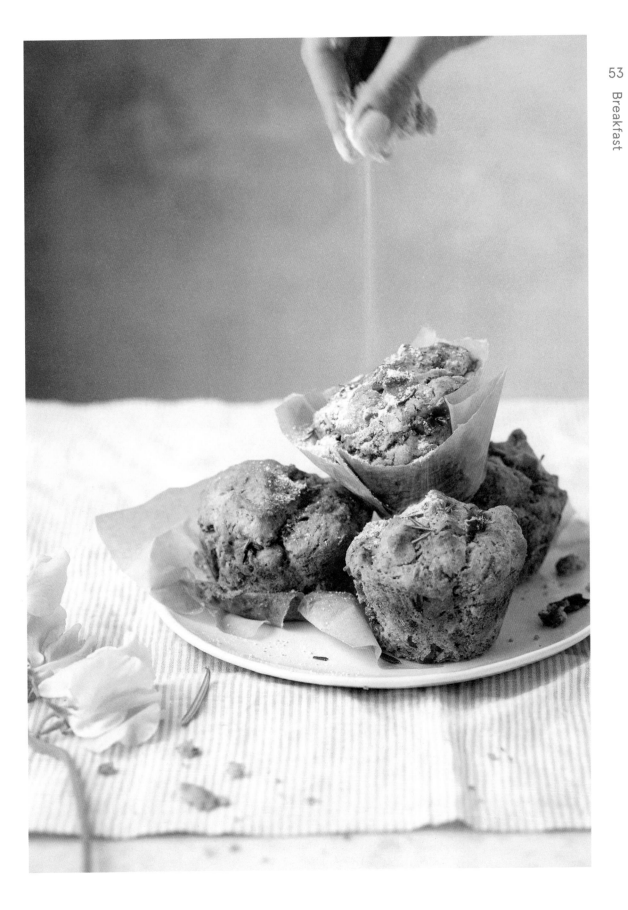

AVOCADO + STRAWBERRY ON RYE

Serves 2

Avocado on toast is one of my favourite weekend breakfast choices when I eat out. It seems to be one of those things that everyone loves. I've livened up my version by adding sweet strawberries and balsamic vinegar.

Ingredients

2 slices of rye bread
8 strawberries, hulled
8–10 mint leaves
1 ripe avocado, stoned
a handful of rocket leaves
balsamic vinegar
freshly ground black pepper

1. Toast the rye bread.
2. Slice the strawberries and roughly chop the mint leaves.
3. Slice or mash the avocado and place on top of the toasted rye bread with the sliced strawberries. Sprinkle over the chopped mint and season with black pepper.
4. Add a handful of rocket leaves, drizzle with balsamic vinegar and dig in.

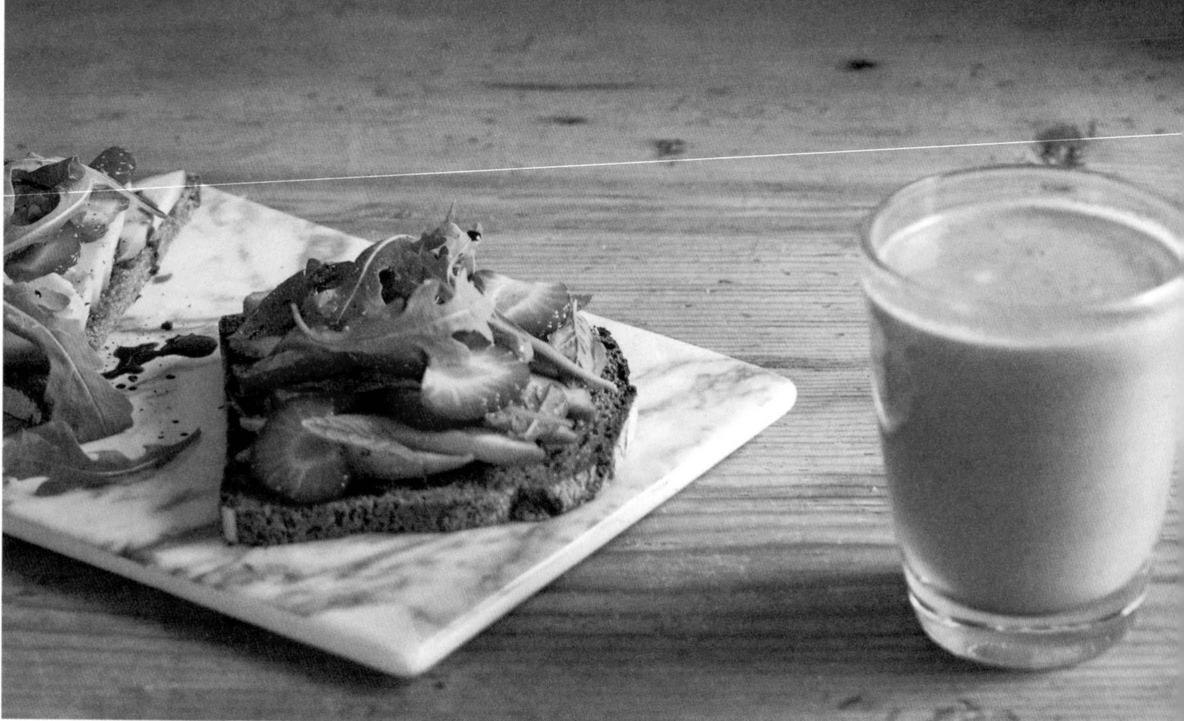

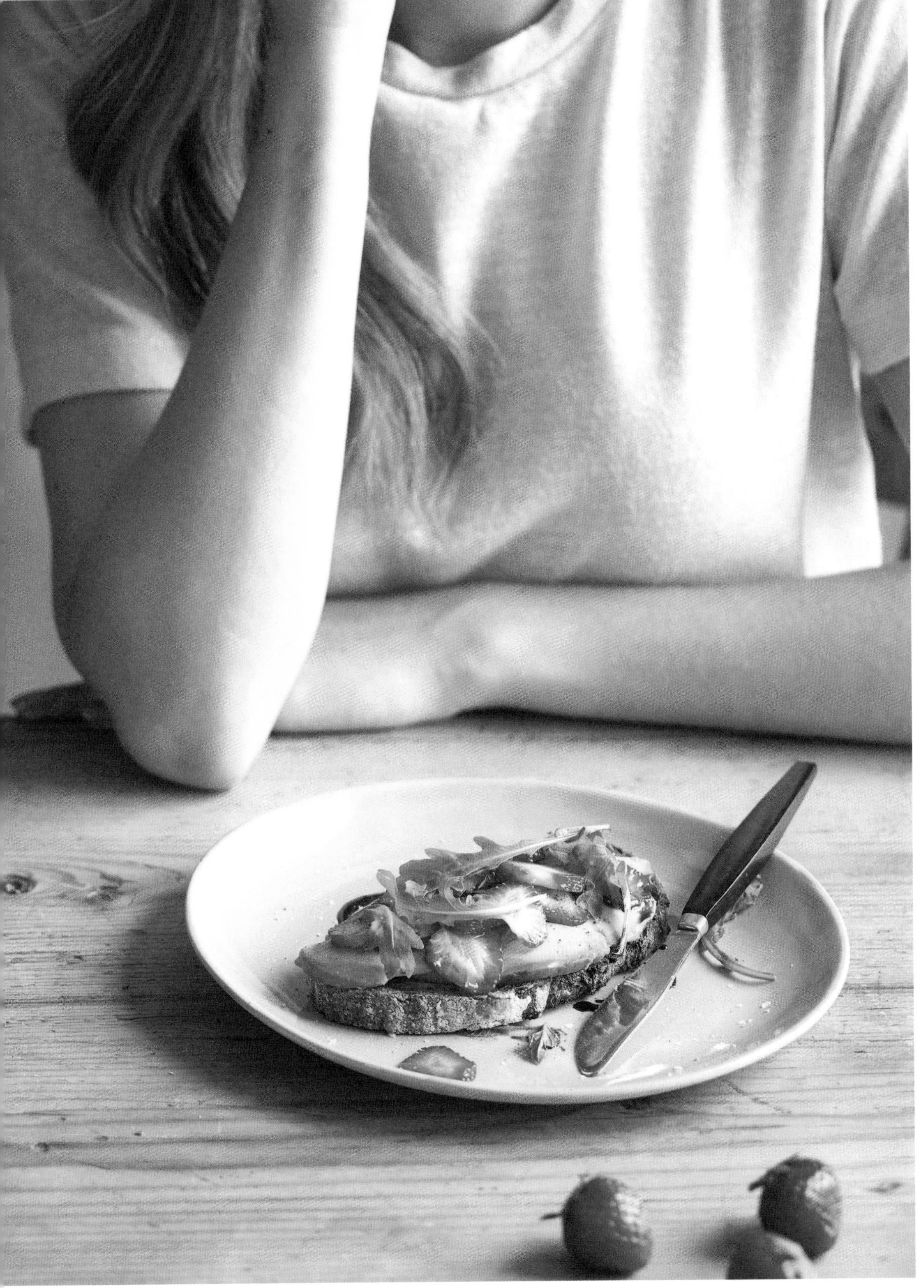

CHIA JAMS

I've never understood why some shop-bought jams are pumped full of additives. Fruits are abundant in bright colours, flavours and contain natural sugars, which means you only need a little natural maple syrup to make the jam lovely and sweet. I love this spread on rye bread or crackers, or stirred into porridge.

STRAWBERRY

Makes approx. 320g

Ingredients

350g (3 cups) strawberries, stalks removed
2 tbsp chia seeds
2 tbsp lemon juice
2 tbsp maple syrup

1. Roughly chop the strawberries and place in a medium saucepan with 2 tablespoons water.
2. Set over a high heat, bring to the boil and turn the heat down to medium-low. Mash the strawberries in the pan with a fork and simmer for 5–7 minutes.
3. Remove from the heat and stir in the chia seeds with the lemon juice and maple syrup. Allow to cool and set for at least 15 minutes before serving. If you prefer a smoother consistency, simply pour into a blender and blend for a few seconds until smooth.
4. Keep in the fridge in an airtight container for up to 2 weeks.

ORANGE + APRICOT

Makes approx. 320g

Ingredients

2 large oranges, peeled
80g (½ cup) fresh apricots
2 tbsp chia seeds
2 tbsp lemon juice
2 tbsp maple syrup

1. Roughly chop the oranges, then halve, destone and roughly chop the apricots.
2. Place in a saucepan over a low-medium heat. Bring to the boil and simmer for 5 minutes.
3. While simmering, use a fork to mash the apricots in the pan.
4. Follow the Strawberry Chia Jam instructions from step 3.

PLUM + GINGER

Makes approx. 320g

Ingredients

350g (2 cups) plums, stoned
5cm piece of fresh ginger, peeled and grated
2 tbsp chia seeds
2 tbsp lemon juice
2 tbsp maple syrup

1. Roughly chop the plums and place in a medium saucepan with 2 tablespoons water.
2. Place over a medium-low heat, bring to the boil, then turn the heat down to low and cover and simmer for 10–15 minutes, until softened.
3. Once softened, use a fork to mash the plums in the pan and add the ginger.
4. Follow the Strawberry Chia Jam instructions from step 3.

Serving ideas ...

Try a teaspoon on top of porridge.
Use as a filling for my Jammy Dodgers (see page 204).
Use as a filling for my Peanut Butter + Jam Flapjacks (see page 221).
Spread onto toasted rye bread for a grab-and-go breakfast.
Spread onto my homemade Oat Cakes (see page 167).

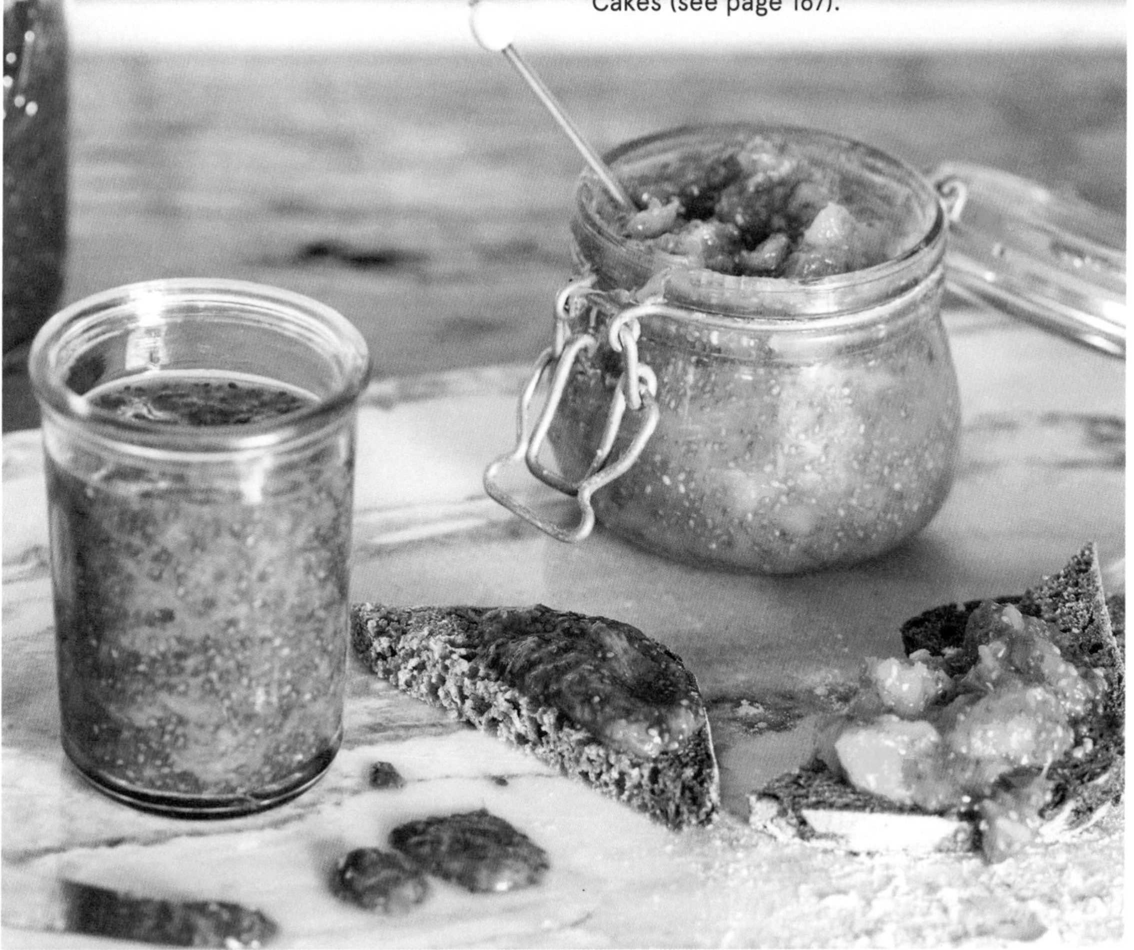

CHOCOLATE PANCAKES WITH RASPBERRY SAUCE

Serves 4

I became incredibly excited when I first discovered I could make delicious pancakes that didn't require eggs or dairy. This is the perfect indulgent breakfast for a special occasion. Whatever the excuse, these will impress your friends and family – see if they even notice that they're healthy, too.

Ingredients

pancake batter

200g (1½ cups) buckwheat flour
375ml (1½ cups) unsweetened almond milk
1 ripe banana, peeled
1 tbsp maple syrup
2 tbsp raw cacao powder
1 heaped tbsp chia seeds
½ tsp bicarbonate of soda
2 tbsp raw cacao nibs
coconut oil

raspberry sauce

150g (1 cup) raspberries
1 tbsp lemon juice
1 tbsp maple syrup
1 tsp plain flour (optional), to thicken

1. Add all the batter ingredients apart from the cacao nibs and coconut oil to a blender and whizz to form a smooth batter. Stir in the cacao nibs and leave to thicken.
2. Put the raspberries, 60ml (¼ cup) water, the lemon juice and maple syrup into a small saucepan and cook over a medium heat, stirring occasionally. When the sauce starts to bubble, turn the heat down to medium and cook for 2–3 minutes until thickened. If it's looking a little too watery, stir in a teaspoon of flour to help the sauce thicken.
3. Heat a little coconut oil in a non-stick frying pan over a medium heat. Once hot, pour about 125ml (½ cup) of the pancake batter into the middle of the pan. Cook for 1–2 minutes on each side and repeat until all the mixture has been used up. You should get 8 pancakes.
4. Stack the pancakes onto plates, drizzle with the delicious raspberry sauce and tuck in!

Serving ideas …

Swap the raspberries in this sauce with blueberries or strawberries and mix and match the pancakes with the sauces.

COCONUT PANCAKES WITH MANGO SAUCE

Serves 4

This is one of my most indulgent breakfast recipes, yet it only calls for ingredients that actually provide a whole bunch of health benefits. I love tropical flavours, so it made sense to combine them with one of my favourite breakfasts. It really is like sunshine on a plate.

Ingredients

mango sauce

1 ripe mango, peeled and stoned
a squeeze of lemon juice

pancake batter

150g (1½ cups) rolled oats
2 ripe bananas, peeled
185ml (1¼ cups) unsweetened almond milk
1 tsp apple cider vinegar
1 tbsp coconut nectar or maple syrup
½ tsp organic vanilla extract
1 tsp bicarbonate of soda
25g (¼ cup) desiccated coconut
coconut oil

topping

1 tbsp desiccated coconut or coconut flakes
a handful of raspberries

1. Start by making the mango sauce. Slice the mango into chunks, add to a blender with 60ml (¼ cup) water and the lemon juice and blend until smooth. Tip into a bowl and keep to one side until ready to serve.
2. Turn the oats into flour by grinding in a blender until fine. Tip into a bowl.
3. Place the bananas, almond milk, apple cider vinegar, coconut nectar and vanilla extract in the blender and whizz until smooth.
4. Add the oat flour and bicarbonate of soda to the banana mixture and blend until smooth. Stir in the desiccated coconut.
5. Heat a little coconut oil in a non-stick frying pan over a medium heat. When the pan is hot, pour an American pancake-sized amount of the mixture - around 60ml (¼ cup) - into the centre of the pan and cook for about 1-2 minutes on each side, until golden and cooked through. Repeat with the remaining mixture until you have 8 pancakes (if you have a large frying pan you can cook 2–3 at a time).
6. Serve the pancakes topped with the mango sauce, desiccated coconut and raspberries.

Tip ... This makes more sauce than needed. It will keep for 2 days in the fridge.

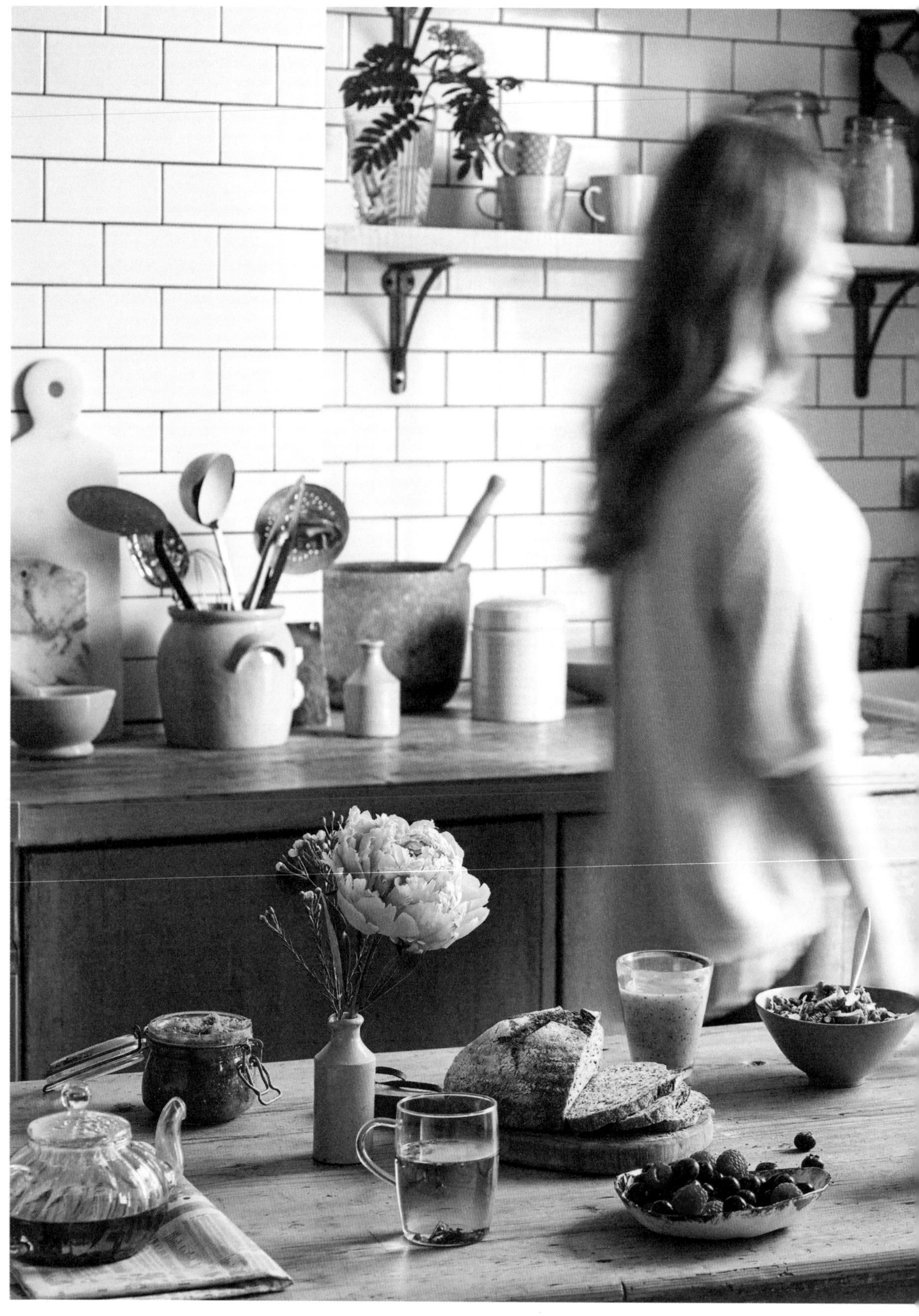

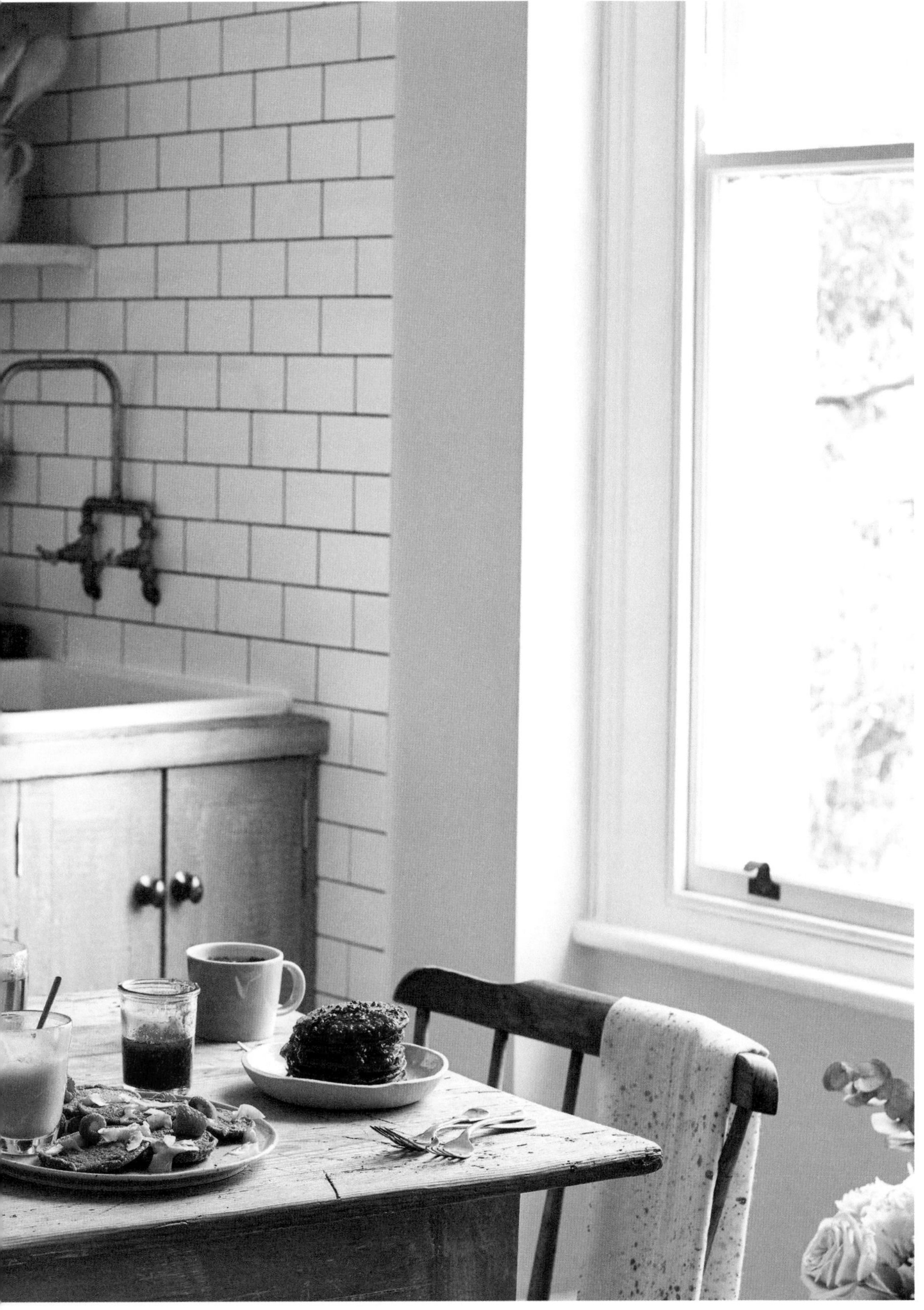

FULL ENGLISH BREAKFAST

Serves 2

One thing that people often ask me is whether I miss out on a full English brekkie, but my version, with garlic mushrooms, grilled vine tomatoes, baked beans and tofu scramble, really hits the spot for a filling, hearty breakfast on a Sunday, after a late one the night before.

Ingredients

grilled tomatoes

250g ripe vine cherry tomatoes
a splash of balsamic vinegar

baked beans

1 x 400g tin cannellini beans, drained
½ tsp onion powder
½ tsp garlic powder
1 x 400g tin passata or sieved tomatoes
1 tsp maple syrup
1 tsp blackstrap molasses
1 garlic clove, peeled and crushed
pink Himalayan salt or sea salt and freshly ground black pepper

garlic mushrooms

1 tbsp coconut oil
10 button mushrooms, halved
2 garlic cloves, peeled and crushed

1. Preheat the grill to medium-high.
2. Put the tofu on a chopping board, place another chopping board on top and place a heavy pan or plate on top to press the tofu down to remove excess water. Leave it while you make the beans and mushrooms.
3. Meanwhile, start by making the beans. Simply add all the ingredients to a small saucepan with a pinch of salt and black pepper. Set over a medium-high heat and bring to the boil. Reduce the heat to medium and simmer for 10 minutes, stirring occasionally.
4. Meanwhile, to make the mushrooms, heat the coconut oil in a small frying pan over a medium heat and fry the mushrooms for 5 minutes until lightly browned and cooked through, stirring occasionally and adding the garlic about a minute before the end.
5. Place the tomatoes (still on their vine) on a baking sheet, sprinkle with sea salt and a little balsamic vinegar and grill for 5-10 minutes, until they start to brown.
6. Once the tofu has been weighed down for 20 minutes, drain any liquid, pat the tofu dry with kitchen paper and cut into cubes.

tofu scramble
½ x 400g pack firm tofu
1 tsp coconut oil
½ tsp turmeric
½ tsp ground cumin
2 tbsp lemon juice
1 tsp nutritional yeast

toasted rye bread, to serve
mashed avocado (optional), to serve

7. To make the scramble, heat the coconut oil in a frying pan over a medium heat. Use your hands to crumble in the tofu, then add the remaining ingredients and cook for about 5 minutes, stirring occasionally.
8. Season to taste and serve everything together with toasted rye bread and mashed avocado, if you like.

Tip ... To save time prepping, you can make the beans in advance and reheat when you are ready to serve.

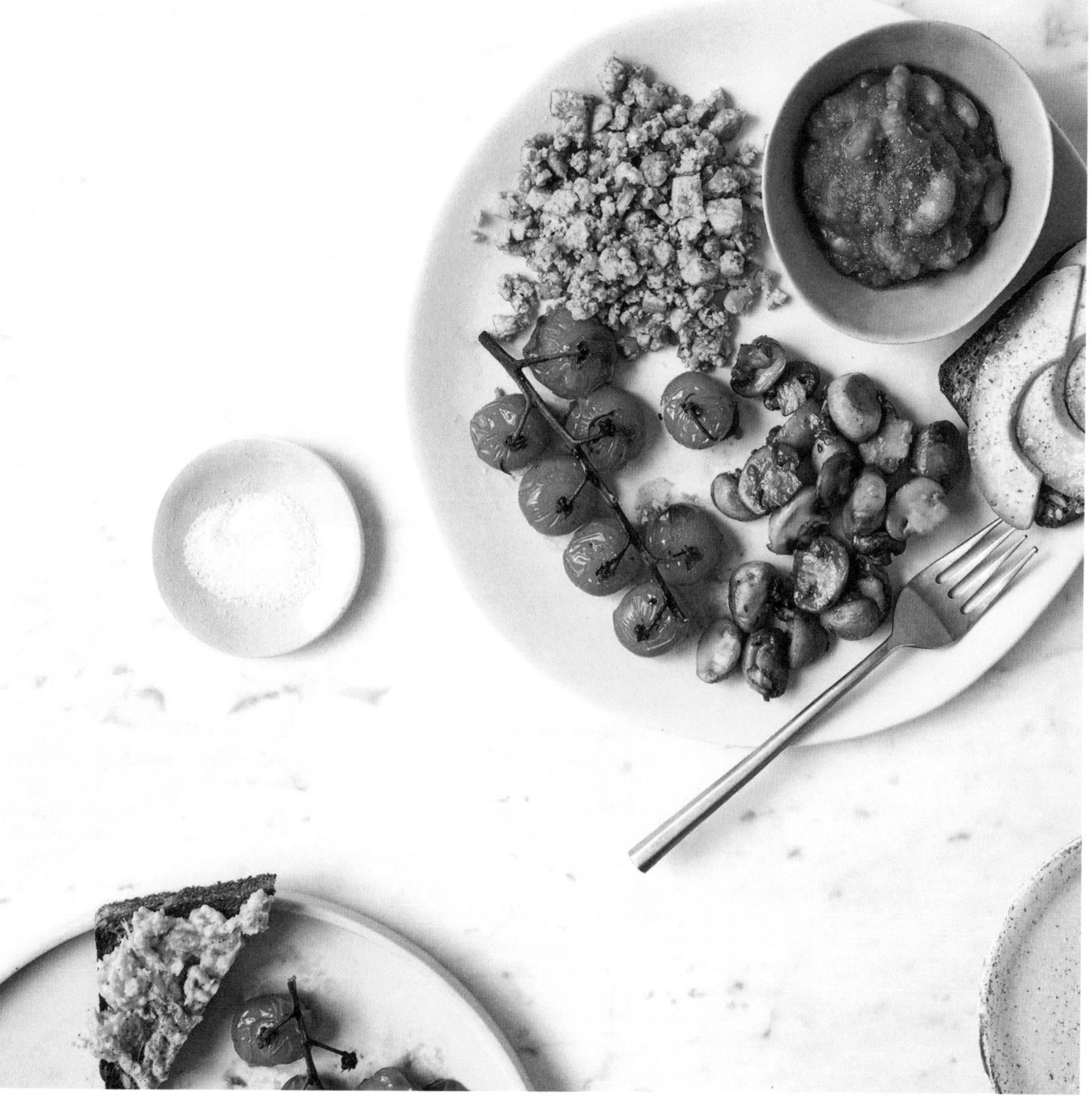

CREAMY MUSHROOMS + BEANS ON TOAST

Serves 2

This is a great breakfast to cook at the weekend when you have a bit more time. Baked beans are such a British comfort food, and incredibly easy to make. I've adapted the traditional method by adding a variety of unconventional flavours, such as garlic, and coconut milk for creaminess.

Ingredients

- 1 tsp coconut oil
- 2 garlic cloves, peeled and thinly sliced
- 2 large ripe vine tomatoes, chopped
- 6 chestnut mushrooms, thinly sliced
- ½ x 400g tin coconut milk
- ½ lemon
- 2 tbsp finely chopped chives, plus extra to serve
- ½ x 400g tin cannellini beans, drained
- 1 tsp paprika
- 2 slices of rye bread
- pink Himalayan salt or sea salt and freshly ground black pepper

1. Heat the oil in a saucepan and fry the garlic and tomatoes for about 3 minutes, stirring occasionally, then add the sliced mushrooms and continue to fry for another 2 minutes, stirring regularly.

2. Pour in the coconut milk, squeeze in the lemon juice and add the chopped chives and beans. Simmer over a medium-high heat for about 8-12 minutes until the sauce has thickened. Season to taste with the paprika, salt and black pepper.

3. Toast the rye bread and pour the creamy mushrooms and beans over the top. Sprinkle with the fresh chives.

Tip ... Keep any leftover lemon to make my Morning Detox Water (see page 231).

CARROT + GINGER GRANOLA BARS

Makes 10

I've always loved the combination of carrot and ginger, whether in a juice, a dessert or a curry! I'm such a grazer, so I love to make things that can go in my handbag and I can grab whenever I'm hungry. These make a lovely, light breakfast option to enjoy on the move.

Ingredients

coconut oil, for greasing
8 medjool dates, pitted
150g (1½ cups) rye flakes
60g (½ cup) pumpkin seeds
100g (1 cup) rolled oats
90g (¾ cup) unsalted raw walnuts, chopped
2 carrots, peeled and finely grated
3cm piece of fresh ginger, peeled and finely grated
3 tsp ground cinnamon
1 tsp turmeric
½ tsp ground nutmeg
60g (½ cup) raisins

1. Preheat the oven to 170°C/325°F/gas 3. Grease a 20cm square baking tin with coconut oil and line with greaseproof paper.
2. Place the dates with 250ml (1 cup) water in a small saucepan over a medium heat and cook for 10 minutes, stirring occasionally.
3. Turn the heat down to low, use a fork to mash the dates in the pan until smooth, then cook for a further 10 minutes, stirring occasionally.
4. Mix together the rye flakes, seeds, oats and walnuts in a large bowl.
5. Stir the carrots and ginger into the date paste with the spices and raisins. Add to the bowl of dry ingredients and mix well.
6. Pour the mixture into the lined baking tray, smoothing down the top with the back of a spoon, and bake for 35 minutes until golden.
7. Allow to cool in the tin for 10 minutes before cutting into 10 rectangles (this will be easier if it's still warm, but not hot). Store in an airtight container.

Tip ... If you don't have any rye flakes, these work just as well if you replace the flakes with extra oats.

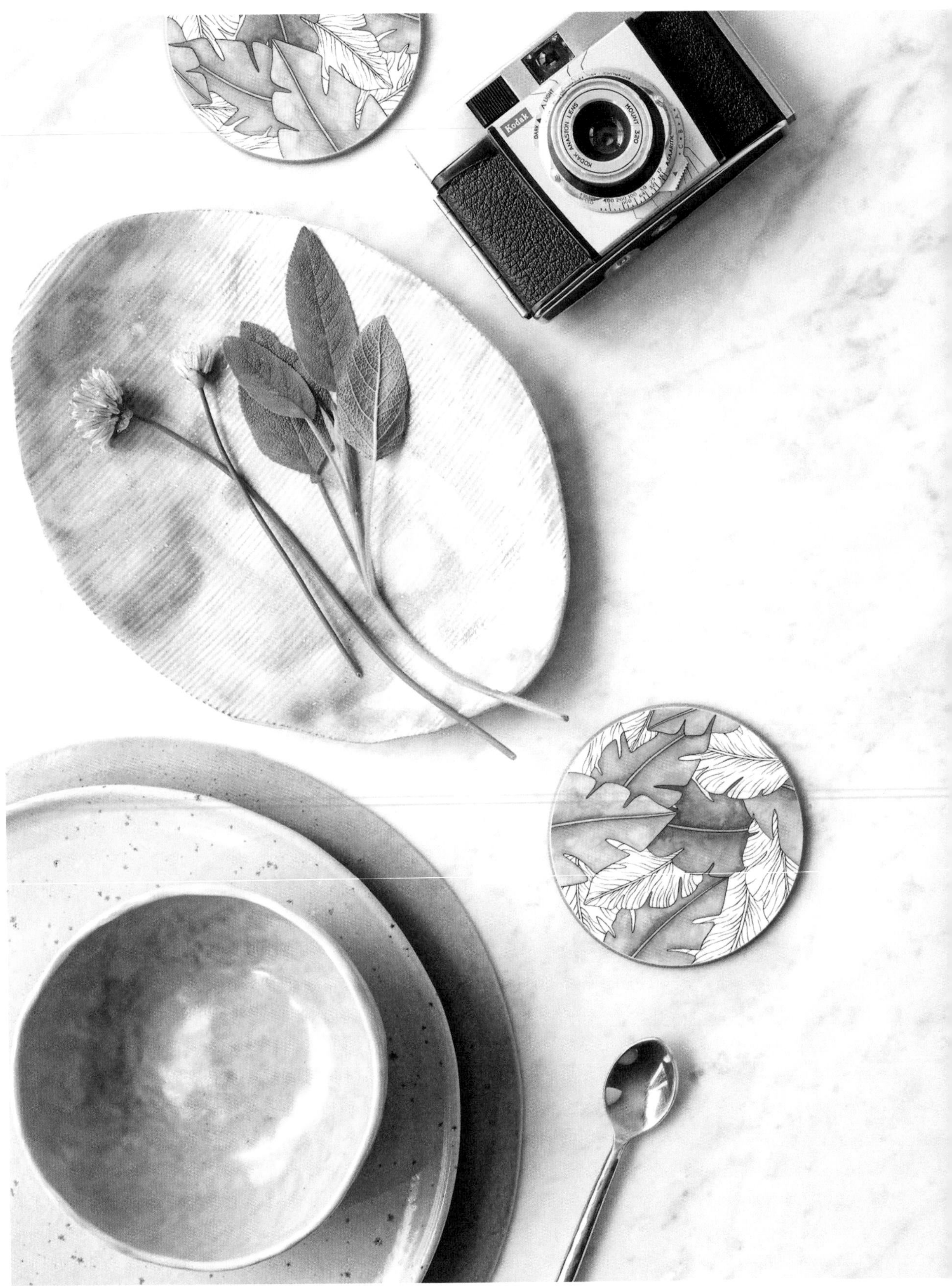
Kodak
KODAK ANASTON LENS
MOUNT 320

Lunch

02

GREEK ISLAND SALAD

Serves 4

My love for Greek salads began on the beautiful island of Santorini, where my friends and I sat around the pool with a large bowl on our laps every day! I've added a few more ingredients to make it a substantial lunch, yet it still transports me back to that Mediterranean sunshine every time I make it.

Ingredients

1 Romaine lettuce, sliced into long strips
1 cucumber, diced
4 large ripe vine tomatoes, diced
1 ripe avocado, peeled, stoned and diced
½ red onion, sliced
10 black olives, pitted and sliced
5 medjool dates, pitted and diced
¼ bunch of fresh mint, leaves picked and chopped
1 x 400g tin of chickpeas, drained
a handful of unsalted raw cashew nuts, chopped
2 tbsp each of pumpkin seeds and hemp seeds (optional)

dressing

a squeeze of lime juice
2 tbsp extra-virgin olive oil
1 tbsp balsamic vinegar

1. Tip everything into a large bowl apart from the cashew nuts and seeds, if using.
2. In a small bowl, mix together a squeeze of lime juice, the olive oil and balsamic vinegar. Pour over the salad and toss to coat.
3. Serve sprinkled with the crushed cashew nuts and seeds, if using.

SPICY ASIAN TOFU SALAD

Serves 2

When I was in Mauritius, there was a place that served an incredible cold tofu salad that I became obsessed with! Those flavours inspired this dish. It's not too often that I include soy products in my food, but the tofu here really pulls the whole dish together.

Ingredients

- ½ x 400g block firm tofu
- 100g buckwheat noodles
- 1 tsp coconut oil
- 1 carrot, peeled
- ¼ red cabbage, thinly sliced
- 2 spring onions, trimmed and sliced
- a handful of beansprouts
- a large bunch of fresh coriander, chopped, with a few leaves reserved to serve
- 2 tbsp unsalted raw peanuts, chopped, to serve
- 1 tsp sesame seeds, to serve

dressing

- juice of 1 lime
- 2 tbsp tamari
- 1 tsp apple cider vinegar
- 1 tbsp sesame oil
- 1 tbsp smooth peanut butter
- ½ fresh red chilli, deseeded and sliced

1. Put the tofu on a chopping board, place another chopping board on top and place a heavy pan or plate on top to press the tofu down to remove excess water. Leave it for about 20 minutes while you cook the noodles.
2. Cook the buckwheat noodles in a pan of boiling water over a medium heat for 12 minutes or according to the packet instructions. Drain, rinse under cold water to separate the noodles and set aside.
3. Once the tofu has been weighed down for 20 minutes, drain any liquid, pat the tofu dry with kitchen paper and cut into cubes.
4. Heat the coconut oil in a frying pan and fry the tofu for 7–10 minutes, stirring occasionally, until golden on all sides.
5. Use a vegetable peeler to peel the carrot into long strips, like ribbons, then mix all the veg and coriander together in a large bowl with the cooled noodles.
6. Make the dressing by combining the lime juice, tamari, vinegar, sesame oil, peanut butter and chilli in a small bowl. Use a fork to whisk it all together.
7. Add the dressing to the salad and stir to coat. Serve topped with the tofu and sprinkled with the chopped peanuts, sesame seeds and coriander leaves.

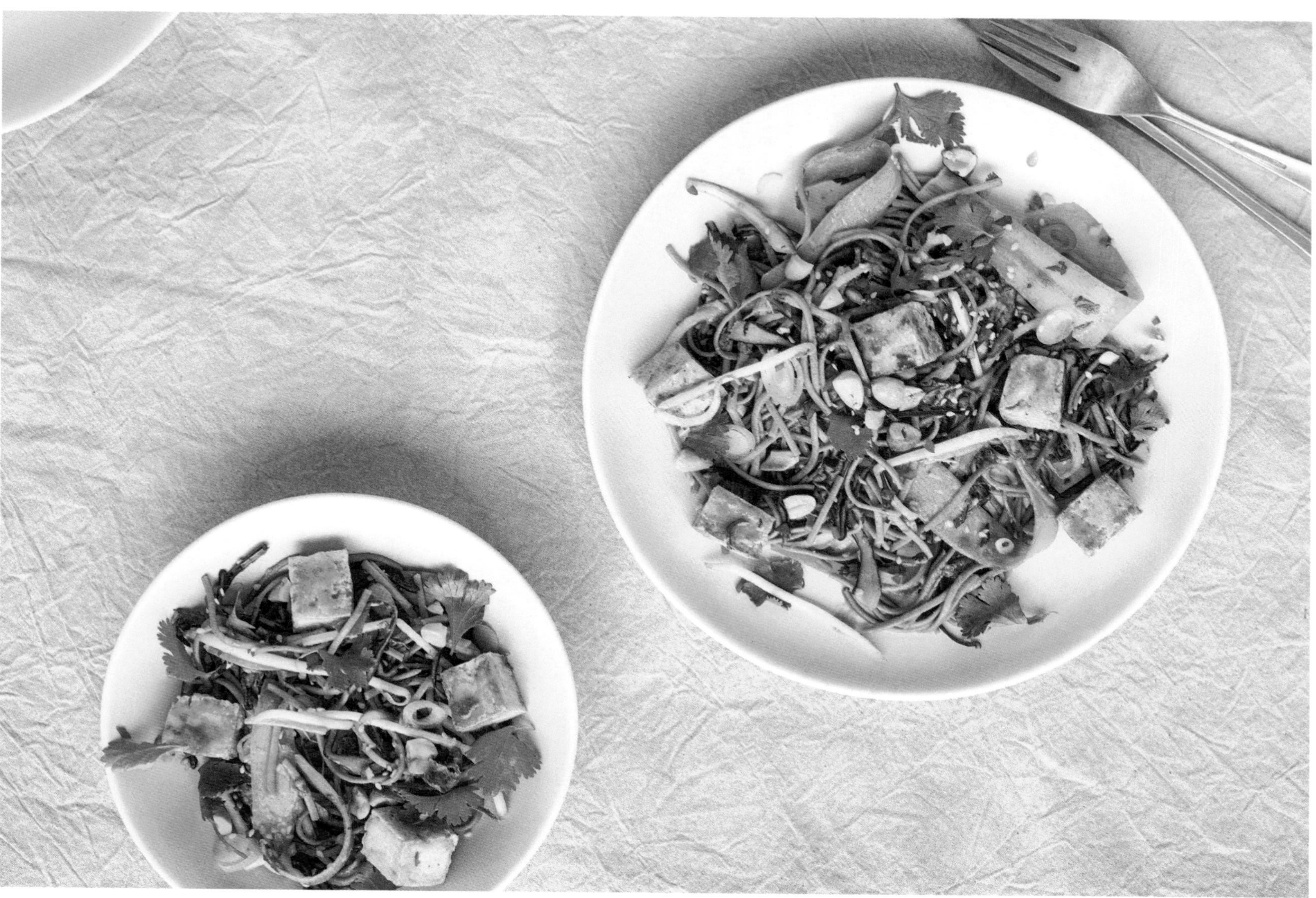

ROASTED FENNEL, LENTIL + FIG SALAD

Serves 2

These flavour combinations are some of my favourites. The distinctive anise taste of fennel and aromatic dill combined with fresh lemon and sweet figs and the delicate crunch of their seeds creates a wonderful, well-rounded salad. The lentils add a real substance to keep you feeling fuller for longer.

Ingredients

100g (½ cup) dried green lentils, rinsed
1 large fennel bulb
olive oil
3 fresh figs, quartered
a small handful of fresh dill, chopped
pink Himalayan salt or sea salt and freshly ground black pepper

dressing

½ lemon
1 tbsp extra-virgin olive oil
½ tsp ground cumin

1. Preheat the oven to 180°C/350°F/gas 4.
2. Place the lentils in a small saucepan, cover with cold water and place over a medium-high heat. Bring to the boil, then turn the heat down to low and simmer for 20 minutes or until cooked through, adding more water if needed. Drain, tip back into the pan and leave to cool.
3. Remove any tatty outer leaves from the fennel, cut into 1cm wedges and place in a roasting tray with a drizzle of olive oil and a pinch of salt and black pepper.
4. Roast in the hot oven for 30-35 minutes, turning halfway to make sure all the wedges are evenly cooked. Remove from the oven and allow to cool.
5. To make the dressing, zest the lemon and set the zest aside. Mix together the extra-virgin olive oil, lemon juice and cumin in a small bowl.
6. Mix the lentils and fennel together with the dressing and serve with the fig quarters, scattering over the chopped dill and a little lemon zest.

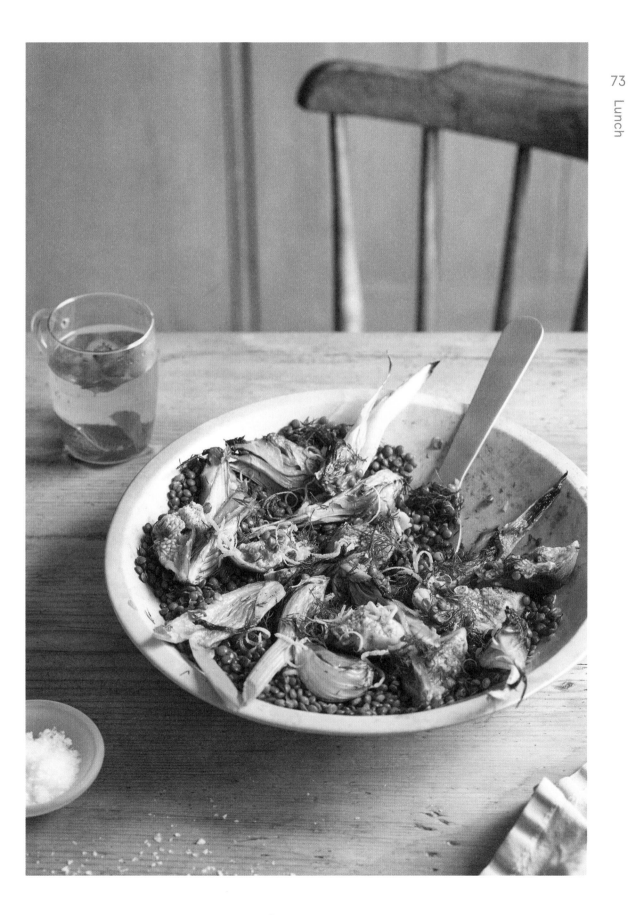

MASSAGED KALE CAESAR SALAD

Serves 2

I used to love Caesar salads but they usually contain little nutritional value, and of course contain heaps of dairy in the dressing. I've 'superfooded' mine to contain an abundance of antioxidants from ingredients such as kale and tahini. What's more, it has a real punch of flavour.

Ingredients

- 1 lemon
- 180g (4 tightly packed cups) curly kale leaves
- 1 tbsp extra-virgin olive oil
- ½ thick slice of rye bread
- 5 unsalted raw cashew nuts, chopped
- 5 black olives, pitted and sliced
- 6 vine cherry tomatoes, quartered (optional)
- pink Himalayan salt or sea salt

dressing

- 1 tbsp capers
- 1 tsp Dijon mustard
- 2 garlic cloves, peeled
- 2 tbsp tahini
- 3 tbsp unsweetened almond milk
- 1 tbsp nutritional yeast
- pink Himalayan salt or sea salt and freshly ground black pepper

1. Zest the lemon and keep to one side. Place the kale in a bowl with the juice of half the lemon, the olive oil and a pinch of salt and rub the kale leaves between your fingers for about 3 minutes until softened and darkened in colour.

2. Add all the dressing ingredients to a small food processor or blender with the juice from the remaining lemon half and a pinch of salt and pepper and whizz until smooth. Stir 3 tablespoons of the dressing into the kale and mix until well coated.

3. To make the croutons, toast the rye bread until nice and crispy (you may need to toast the bread twice).

4. Cut the toasted rye bread into small cubes and serve scattered over the dressed kale with the chopped cashews, sliced olives, lemon zest and the cherry tomatoes, if using.

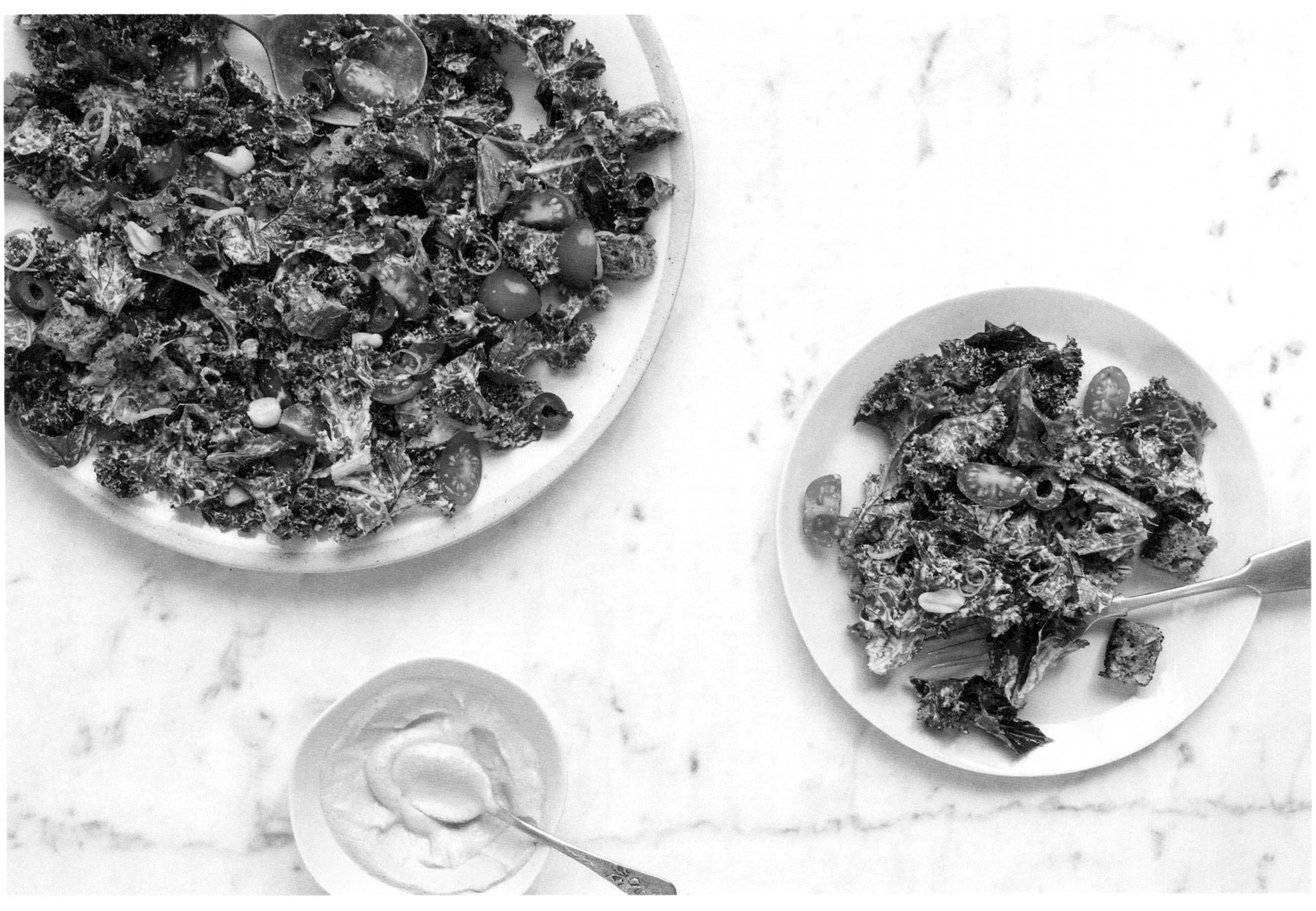

GRAIN SALADS – 3 WAYS

Grains make the perfect salad for summer – ideal for picnics! These are easy recipes using super healthy quinoa, pearl barley and bulgur wheat, with lots of fresh herbs, vegetables and spices for flavour. They make a lovely alternative to rice salads, and are also great as side dishes.

ROASTED ASPARAGUS + BEETROOT SALAD WITH PEARL BARLEY

Serves 2

Ingredients

2 beetroots (about 160g)
50g (¼ cup) pearl barley, rinsed
4 asparagus spears
olive oil
2 large handfuls of watercress
4 unsalted raw Brazil nuts, chopped
pink Himalayan salt or sea salt and freshly ground black pepper

dressing

2 tbsp balsamic vinegar
2 tbsp extra-virgin olive oil
juice of ½ orange
pink Himalayan salt or sea salt and freshly ground black pepper

1. Preheat the oven to 200°C/400°F/gas 6.
2. Trim the ends off the beetroots, wrap each one in tin foil and bake in the hot oven for 40 minutes.
3. Place the barley in a saucepan with 375ml (1½ cups) cold water. Cover, bring to the boil and simmer over a medium heat for 40 minutes or according to packet instructions until soft, then set aside to cool.
4. Slice the woody ends off the asparagus and thinly slice lengthways into long, thin ribbons. Rub with a small amount of olive oil, salt and black pepper and lay on a baking tray. Cook in the oven with the beetroot for the last 10 minutes, turning halfway through.
5. Allow the beetroot to cool, then peel off the skin and slice into eighths.
6. To make the dressing, place the ingredients in a glass and whisk with a fork.
7. Use a fork to fluff up the pearl barley and serve spooned over the watercress. Add the roasted beetroot and asparagus and drizzle over the dressing with a handful of chopped Brazil nuts.

Tip ... Use golden or pink beetroots here if you can get them. They taste beautiful.

BULGUR WHEAT TABBOULEH

Serves 2

Ingredients

40g (¼ cup) bulgur wheat
a small handful of kale, chopped
a couple of sprigs of fresh mint, leaves picked and finely chopped
½ bunch of fresh parsley, leaves picked and finely chopped
2 large ripe vine tomatoes, diced
1 spring onion, finely sliced
½ cucumber, sliced lengthways into eighths and chopped
½ lemon
1 tbsp extra-virgin olive oil
¼ pomegranate, seeded
pink Himalayan salt or sea salt and freshly ground black pepper

1. Cook the bulgur wheat according to the packet instructions, then drain and leave to cool in a serving bowl.
2. Once cool, mix in all the chopped vegetables and herbs. Zest the lemon half and set the zest aside. Squeeze the juice into the bowl with the olive oil and season with salt and black pepper.
3. Sprinkle over the lemon zest and pomegranate seeds and serve.

Tip ... To remove pomegranate seeds I tend to use the water method – cut the pomegranate in half, add to a bowl of water and break apart with your hands to remove the seeds.

AVOCADO + TURMERIC SALAD WITH QUINOA

Serves 2

Ingredients

150g (¾ cup) quinoa, rinsed
1 avocado, peeled and stoned
40g (¼ cup) sun-dried tomatoes, in oil
1 tsp turmeric
¼ tsp ground cumin
a pinch of cayenne pepper
¼ bunch fresh coriander, leaves picked and chopped
a squeeze of lime juice
pink Himalayan salt or sea salt and freshly ground black pepper

1. Tip the quinoa into a saucepan with 375ml (1½ cups) water. Place over a medium heat, bring to the boil, then turn the heat down to low and simmer for 15 minutes until the water has been absorbed and the quinoa is cooked, adding more water if needed. Keep to one side to cool.
2. Chop the avocado into chunks. Rinse the oil off the sun-dried tomatoes and slice into strips.
3. When the quinoa has cooled, fluff up with a fork and stir in the spices. Stir in most of the coriander, avocado and sun-dried tomatoes and add a squeeze of lime juice.
4. Taste and season if needed, then serve scattered with the remaining coriander leaves.

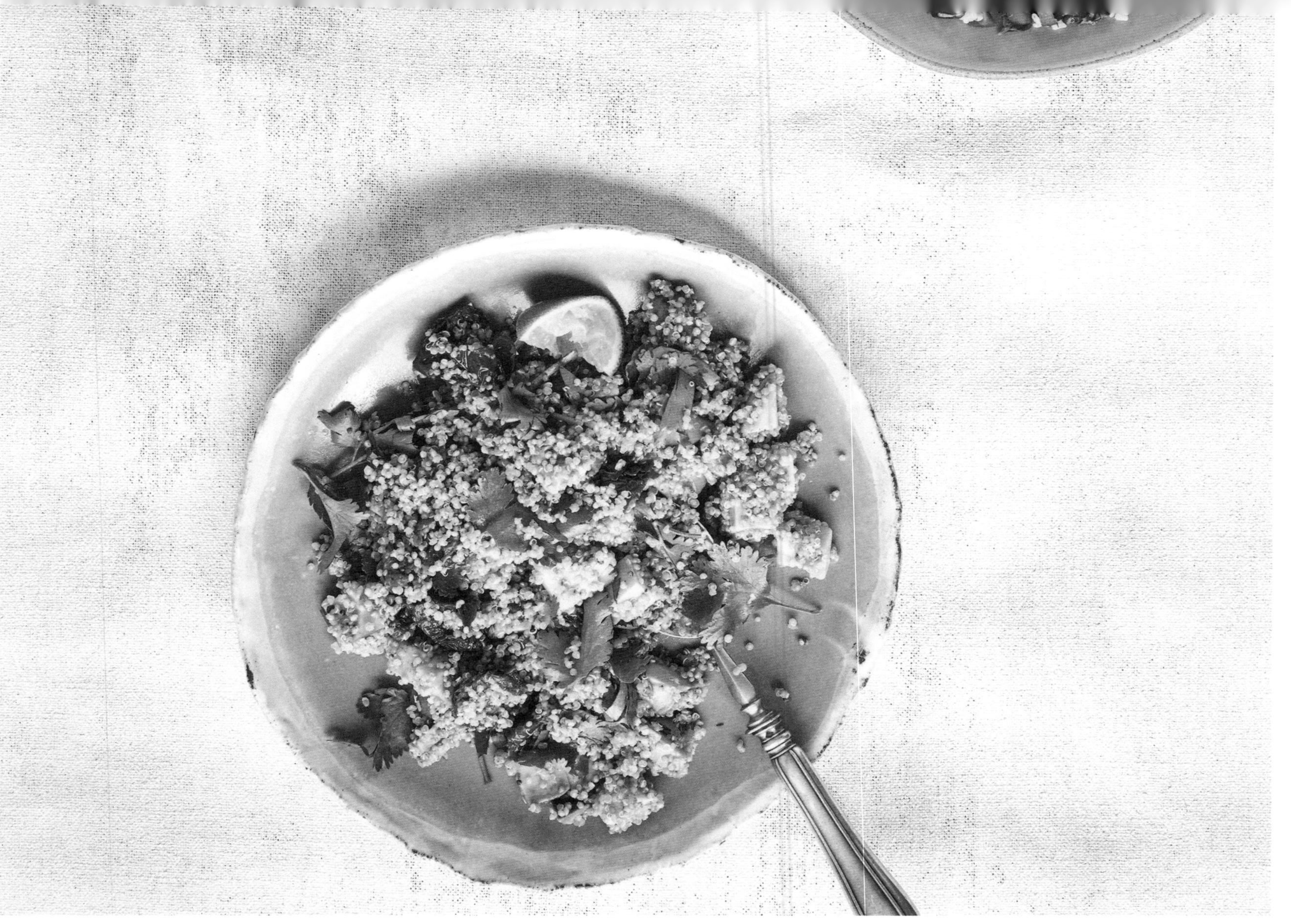

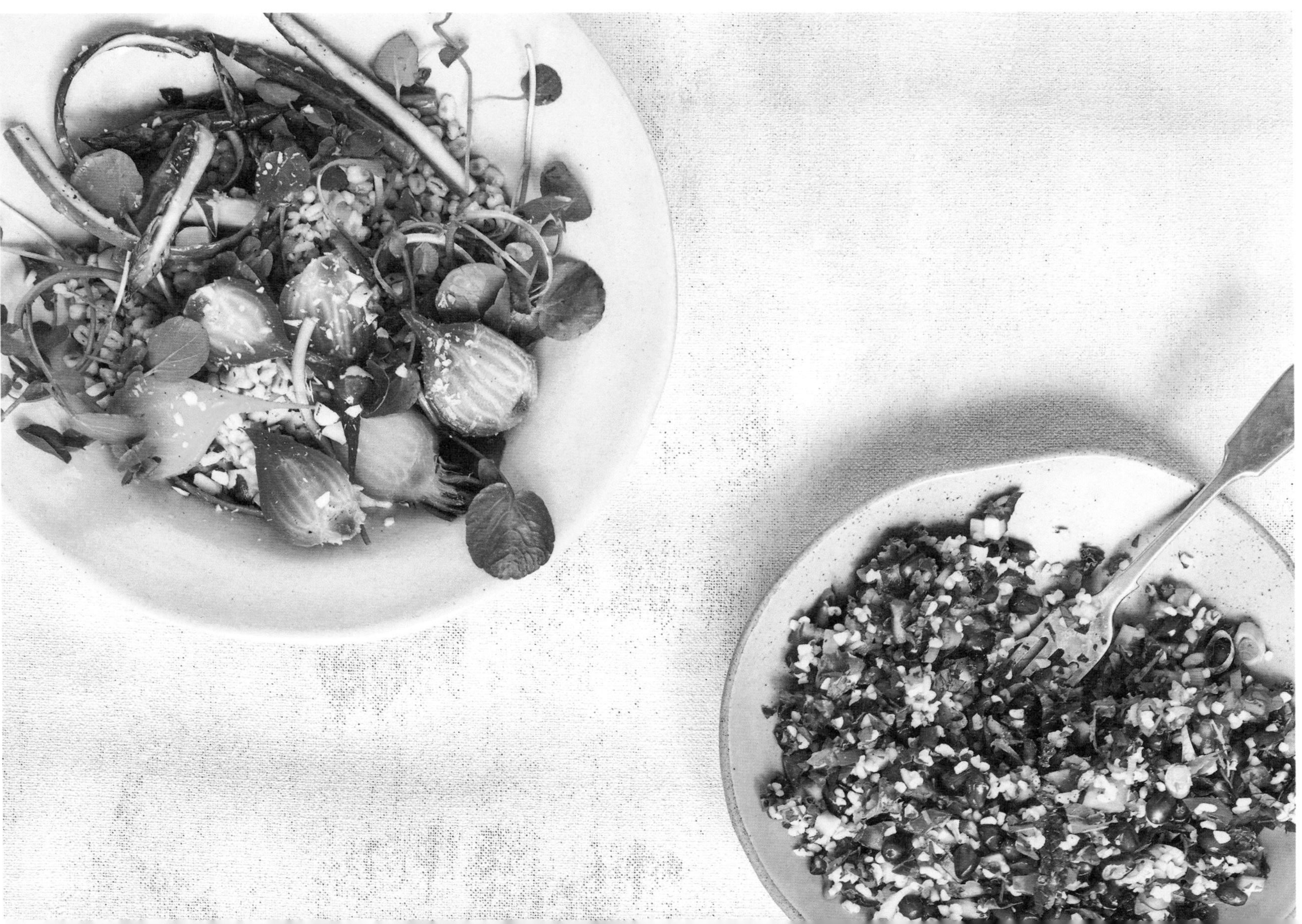

WARMING SQUASH SOUP

Serves 4

This soup is the ultimate winter warmer. When it's frosty outside I love to snuggle up on my sofa with a thick-knitted blanket and a bowl of this. This soup is deliciously creamy from the coconut milk and full of flavour from the herbs and fresh vegetables with a hint of spiciness.

Ingredients

- 1 tsp coconut oil
- 1 onion, diced
- 1 garlic clove, peeled and crushed
- ½ fresh red chilli, deseeded and chopped
- 1 tsp ground cumin
- 1 tsp dried thyme
- ½ tsp ground coriander
- 1 small butternut squash, peeled and chopped
- 2 carrots, peeled and chopped
- ½ x 400g tin coconut milk
- pink Himalayan salt or sea salt and freshly ground black pepper
- a handful of coriander leaves, to serve

1. Heat the coconut oil in a large saucepan over a medium-low heat and gently fry the diced onion for about 5 minutes.
2. Add the garlic, chilli, cumin, thyme and coriander and fry for another minute. Pour in 1.25 litres (5 cups) boiling water, add the squash, carrots and most of the coconut milk and simmer for about 20 minutes or until the vegetables have softened.
3. Season with salt and black pepper and whizz in a blender until smooth. Serve sprinkled with fresh coriander leaves and a drizzle of the remaining coconut milk.

Tip ... My soups serve 4 people, so when I'm cooking just for me I make a batch and freeze the portions I don't need.

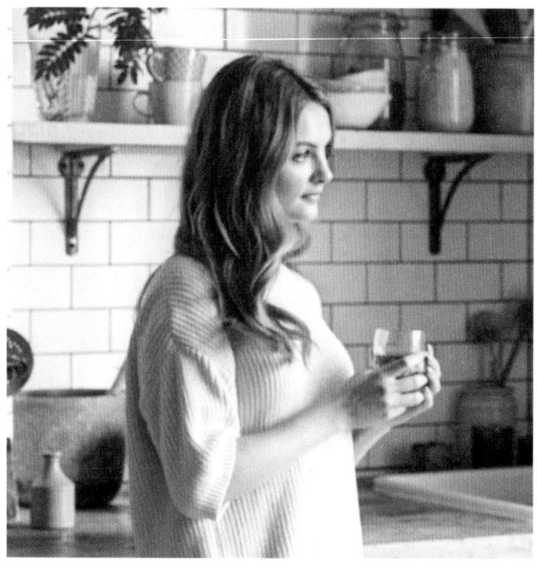

KALE MINESTRONE

Serves 4

It can be hard to find simple plant-based food in Italy, but I love the flavours of that country, so I decided to create a comforting minestrone soup using spelt pasta and kale. For me, every meal should be packed with ingredients that will do our bodies good, which is why I included a dark leafy green here.

Ingredients

1 onion, diced
1 tbsp olive oil
2 garlic cloves, crushed
2 carrots, peeled and diced
2 celery sticks, chopped
1 yellow pepper, deseeded and diced
1 tsp dried oregano
1 organic low-salt vegetable stock cube
1 x 400g tin cannellini beans, drained
2 x 400g tins chopped tomatoes
1 tbsp tomato purée
175g spelt spaghetti
150g tightly packed (2 cups) kale leaves
pink Himalayan salt or sea salt and freshly ground black pepper
a small handful of fresh basil leaves, chopped, to serve

1. Start by frying the onion in the olive oil in a large saucepan over a medium heat for 5-7 minutes until softened.
2. Add the garlic, carrots, celery and pepper and fry for a further 5 minutes. Add a pinch of salt and black pepper with the oregano.
3. Dissolve the stock cube in 500ml (2 cups) boiling water and pour it into the saucepan with the beans, tinned tomatoes and tomato purée. Bring to the boil and simmer for 40 minutes.
4. Snap the spaghetti into 2-3cm pieces, add to the pan and continue to simmer for a further 10 minutes, adding 250-500ml (1-2 cups) more water if needed.
5. Now stir in the kale and simmer for a further 5 minutes.
6. Serve sprinkled with the fresh basil.

Tip ... To make this gluten-free, simply swap the spelt spaghetti for your favourite gluten-free pasta – I love brown rice penne.

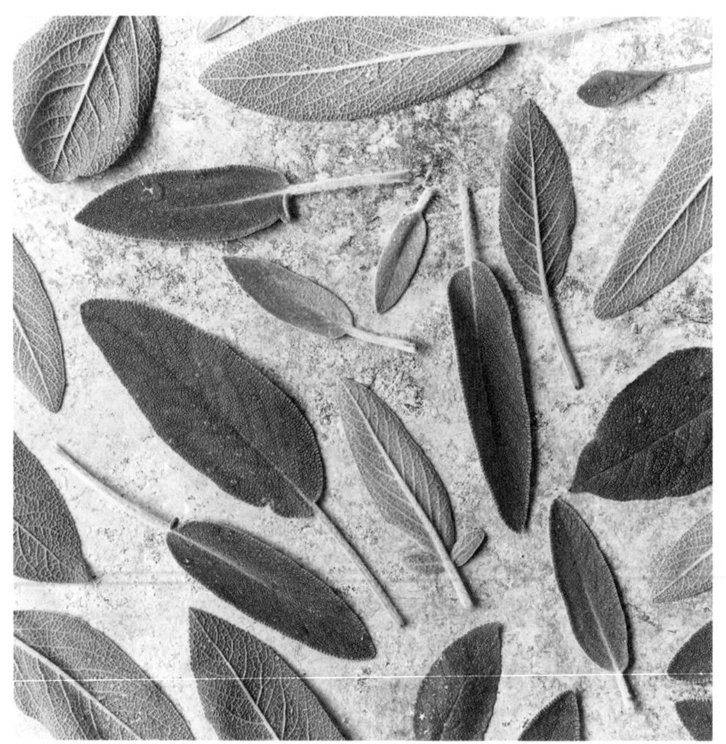

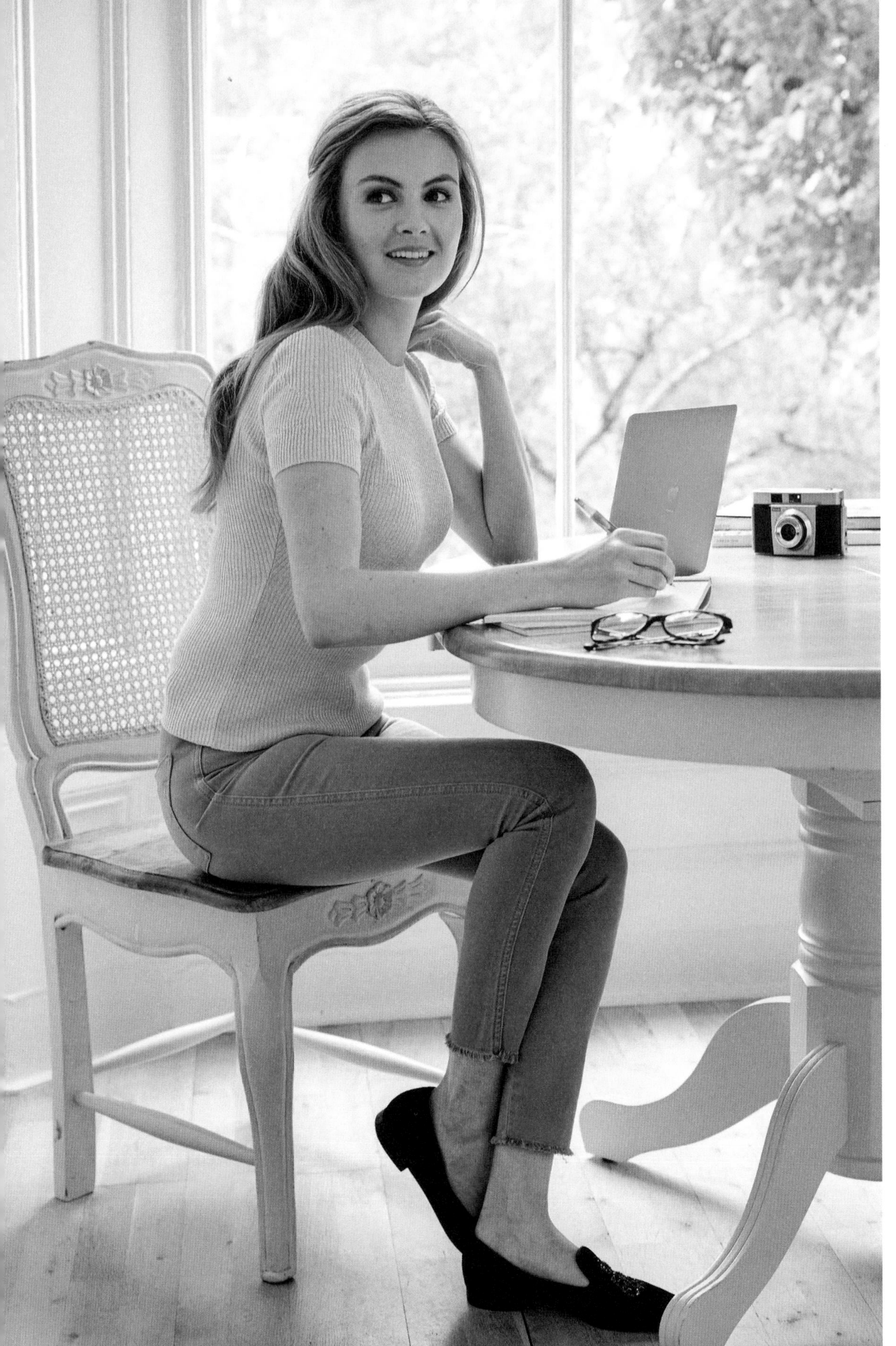

SWEETCORN CHOWDER IN SPELT SOURDOUGH

Serves 4

On a visit to San Francisco in 2013, I tried the famous clam chowder that's served in a sourdough bread bowl. This is my healthy version. It's totally carbolicious, but it's a showstopper presented in the sourdough. Once you're halfway through the soup, break off the bread and dip it in.

Ingredients

- 1 organic low-salt vegetable stock cube
- 150ml (⅔ cup) oat milk or other non-dairy milk
- 60ml (¼ cup) white wine
- 2 medium potatoes, peeled and diced
- 1 tsp coconut oil
- 1 onion, diced
- 1 leek, trimmed and chopped
- 3 garlic cloves, peeled and finely chopped
- 2 sprigs of fresh thyme, leaves picked
- 1 tbsp wholewheat flour
- 1 celery stalk, trimmed and diced
- 2 corn on the cobs
- a squeeze of lemon juice
- pink Himalayan salt or sea salt and freshly ground black pepper
- 4 small round spelt or wholewheat sourdough loaves, to serve
- a couple of sprigs of fresh parsley, leaves picked and chopped, to serve

1. Pour 500ml (2 cups) water into a large saucepan and crumble in the stock cube. Add the oat milk, wine and potatoes. Set over a medium-high heat, bring to the boil, then simmer for 15-20 minutes until the potatoes are just cooked.
2. Meanwhile, heat the coconut oil in a frying pan over a medium-high heat and fry the onion, leek and garlic with the thyme leaves for a few minutes until softened.
3. Stir in the flour to coat the vegetables, then add to the saucepan along with the celery.
4. Slice the kernels off the cobs and add the corn to the pan. Season with a decent amount of salt and black pepper and add a squeeze of lemon juice. Simmer for a further 5 minutes, then remove from the heat.
5. Cut a circle out of the top of the bread loaves and scoop out the bread from the inside to make them hollow.
6. Serve the chowder in the bread bowls and sprinkle over the fresh parsley.

Tip ... If you can't find the right size sourdough roll, simply serve in a bowl with a slice of nice sourdough on the side.

FARMHOUSE VEGETABLE SOUP

Serves 4

Ideally this soup would be made in a rustic farmhouse kitchen using vegetables from the veg patch, but unfortunately this is hugely unrealistic for me living in London, and probably for most of you, too. Nonetheless, we can still get the same flavours with a few simple fresh ingredients.

Ingredients

1 tbsp coconut oil
3 carrots, peeled and chopped
2 celery sticks, chopped
2 leeks, trimmed and chopped
1 potato (about 200g), peeled and chopped
1 parsnip, peeled and chopped
1 small head of broccoli, chopped
1 organic low-salt vegetable stock cube
100g (½ cup) pearl barley, rinsed
2 bay leaves
3 sprigs of fresh thyme
pink Himalayan salt or sea salt and freshly ground black pepper

1. Heat the oil in a large saucepan over a medium-high heat and fry all the vegetables for about 10 minutes, until softened, stirring often and adding a splash of water if the vegetables are catching.
2. Dissolve the stock cube in 1 litre (4 cups) boiling water and pour into the pan with the pearl barley, bay leaves, thyme sprigs and a pinch of salt and pepper.
3. Cover and simmer for 30–40 minutes, or until the barley is soft. Remove the bay leaves and thyme sprigs and serve.

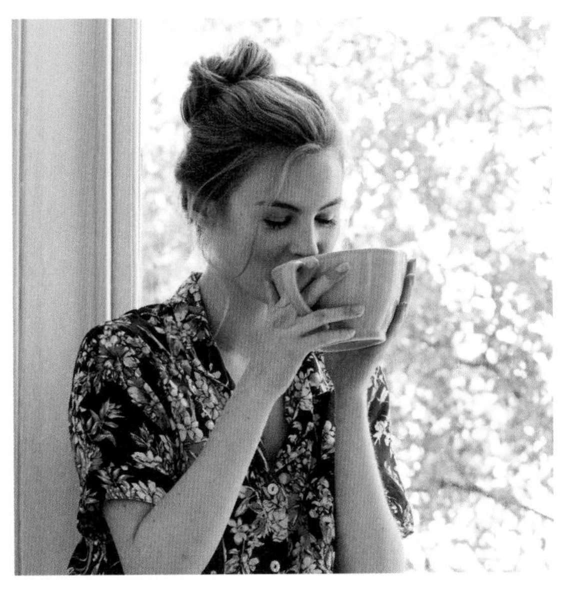

CREAMY CARROT SOUP WITH ROASTED BROCCOLI

Serves 4

One of my favourite lunch choices, soup is quick and easy to make and a great way to get an abundance of nutritious vegetables into your diet. This carrot soup is creamy and velvety smooth, and when paired with the fiery garlic-roasted broccoli it all comes to life.

Ingredients

2 tbsp coconut oil
½ head of broccoli, chopped into florets
4 tbsp lemon juice
1 tsp dried chilli flakes
4 garlic cloves, peeled and finely chopped
2 onions, diced
4 large carrots, peeled and sliced into discs
¼ bunch of fresh thyme, leaves picked
1 tsp paprika
1 litre (4 cups) unsweetened almond milk
pink Himalayan salt or sea salt and freshly ground black pepper

1. Preheat the oven to 200°C/400°F/gas 6.
2. Place half the coconut oil in a large roasting tray and place in the oven for a few seconds to melt. Add the broccoli, toss with the lemon juice and chilli flakes and roast for 15 minutes, stirring and adding two-thirds of the garlic halfway through.
3. Heat the remaining coconut oil in a large saucepan over a medium-low heat. Add the onions and fry for 3-5 minutes. Add the remaining garlic and fry for a further minute.
4. Add the carrots and cook for 6 minutes, then stir in the thyme leaves with the paprika. Pour in 500ml (2 cups) water with the almond milk. Turn the heat up to medium-high, bring to the boil, then simmer uncovered for about 15 minutes until the carrots have softened.
5. Taste and season with salt and black pepper, then place in a blender and whizz until totally smooth.
6. Reheat in the saucepan, if necessary, then serve with the roasted broccoli and garlic sprinkled on top.

GAZPACHO

Serves 2

I spent a lot of my childhood in the Costa Del Sol, in Spain, with family, and an ongoing joke whenever we're there is that we all order the same thing at lunch: a bowl of gazpacho. My version of this smooth, chilled vegetable soup is so refreshing in the summer heat and is packed with flavour.

Ingredients

1 cucumber, roughly chopped
10 ripe vine tomatoes, quartered
1 red pepper, deseeded and roughly chopped
½ green pepper, deseeded and roughly chopped
3 garlic cloves, peeled and roughly chopped
½ onion, roughly chopped
1 tbsp apple cider vinegar or lemon juice
60ml (¼ cup) extra-virgin olive oil
¼–½ tsp cayenne pepper

1. Add all the vegetables to a blender, reserving a small chunk each of cucumber, pepper and onion.
2. Add the vinegar, olive oil, cayenne pepper and 250ml (1 cup) water and blend until smooth.
3. Sieve the gazpacho into a large bowl or jug, using a wooden spoon to press the soup through the sieve if it slows down.
4. Place in the fridge to chill for at least 3 hours.
5. Finely dice the reserved cucumber, pepper and onion.
6. Once cooled, serve the gazpacho in bowls sprinkled with the diced veg.

Tip ... If you have an extractor juicer, blend the gazpacho ingredients in this and skip step 3.

RAW PEA + COURGETTE SOUP

Serves 2

I made this raw soup for my first ever food demonstration. You may be wary about a raw green soup, but trust me on this one! It's so simple to make, it doesn't require any more effort than making a smoothie. Serve this cold to keep the nutrient value as high as possible.

Ingredients

75g (½ cup) frozen peas
½ courgette
1 ripe avocado, peeled and stoned
1 spring onion, trimmed
1 garlic clove, peeled
2 tbsp lemon juice
5 fresh mint leaves, plus extra to serve
¼ tsp cayenne pepper, plus a pinch to serve
pink Himalayan salt or sea salt and freshly ground black pepper
1 tbsp flaked almonds, to serve

1. Place all the ingredients except for the almonds into a blender that works with ice, if using frozen peas, along with 250ml (1 cup) water, and whizz until totally smooth and creamy, adding more water if you prefer it a little looser.

2. Season to taste and serve sprinkled with the flaked almonds, extra mint leaves and cayenne pepper.

Tip ... Spring Garden Risotto (see page 144), is a delicious recipe for using up the leftover courgette.

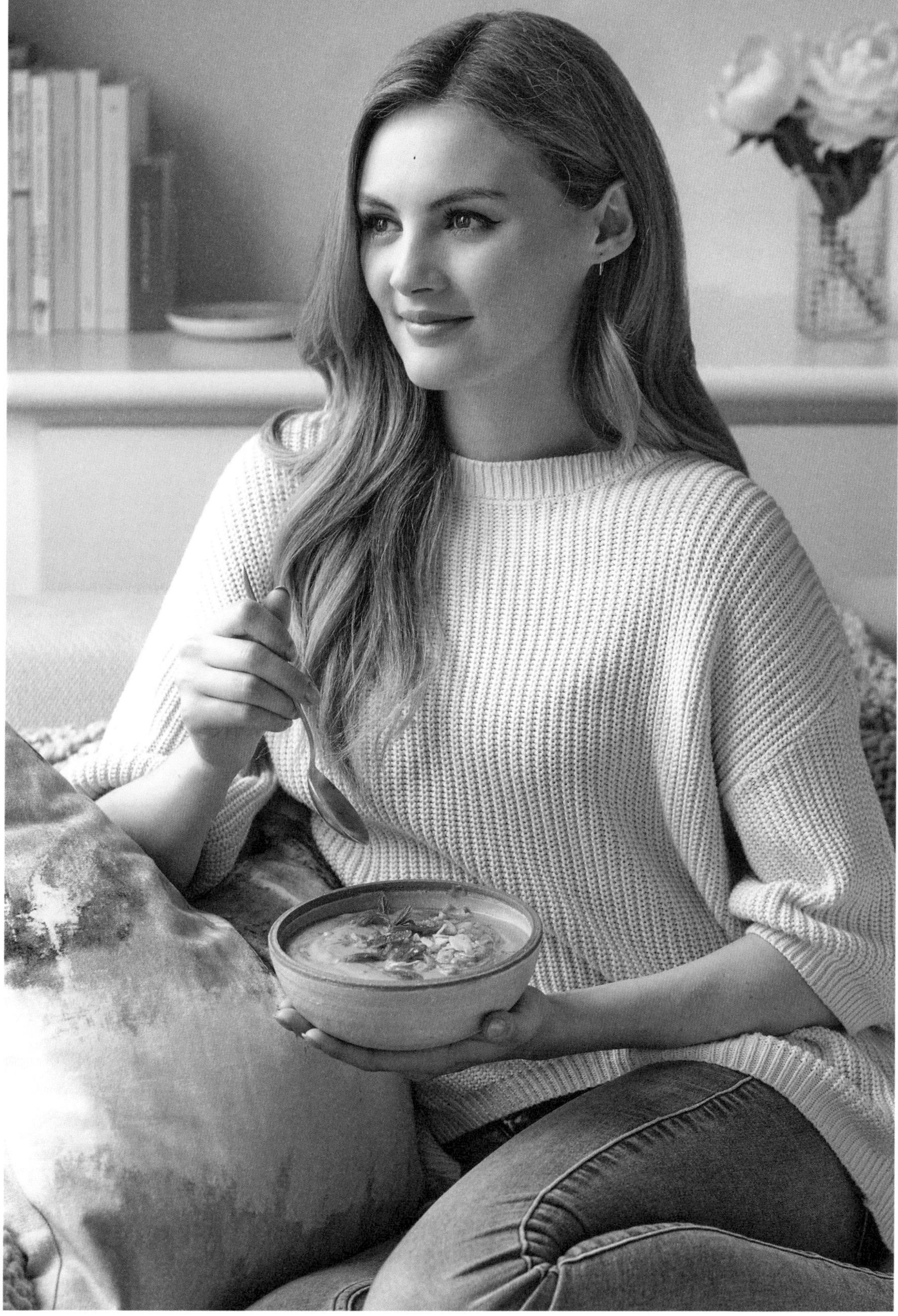

CHINESE CAULIFLOWER RICE WITH PAK CHOY

Serves 4

One of my old guilty pleasures was Chinese special fried rice ordered from the local take-away. I loved it. That's what inspired me to make this Asian lunchtime dish full of goodness; I find rice to be quite heavy sometimes, so when I fancy something light, cauliflower is a great alternative.

Ingredients

cauliflower rice

- 1 head of cauliflower, quartered
- 1 tbsp flaked almonds
- 1 tbsp desiccated coconut
- 1 tbsp sesame oil
- 1 garlic clove, peeled and crushed
- 1 fresh red chilli, deseeded and chopped
- 2 tbsp tamari
- ½ tsp ground cinnamon
- 3cm piece of fresh ginger, peeled and chopped
- ½ onion, peeled and chopped
- 1 x 190g tin sweetcorn, drained
- 200g (1½ cups) frozen peas
- a handful of beansprouts
- ¼ bunch of fresh coriander, leaves picked, to serve

1. Grate the cauliflower on a box grater, or pulse in a food processor until it forms a consistency similar to rice.
2. In a small dry frying pan over a medium-high heat, toast the flaked almonds for a minute or two, tossing often until lightly browned and adding the desiccated coconut halfway. Toss often (it's easy to burn these, so keep an eye on them!). Tip onto a plate and set aside.
3. Place a wok or large frying pan over a medium heat, add the sesame oil and fry the garlic, chilli, tamari, cinnamon, ginger and onion for a couple of minutes, stirring.
4. Now add the cauliflower rice, sweetcorn and peas. Stir until all the ingredients are mixed together and cook for about 10–15 minutes, adding the beansprouts for the last 5 minutes, stirring often.
5. While the rice is cooking, make the pak choy. Heat the coconut oil in a large frying pan or wok on a medium heat. Add the broccoli and cook for 5–7 minutes, stirring, until it is cooked but still has a bit of bite, then remove to a plate.

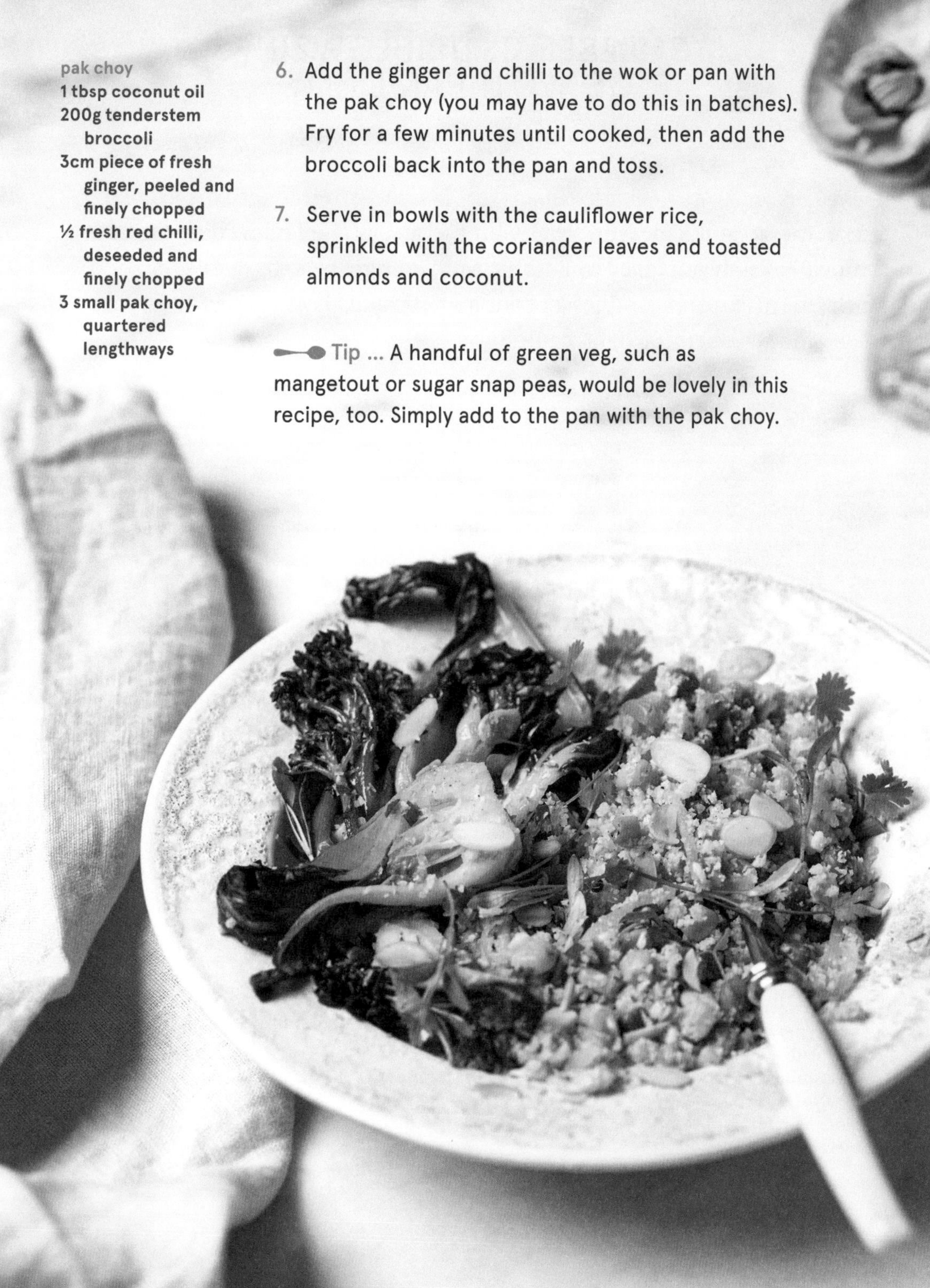

pak choy
1 tbsp coconut oil
200g tenderstem broccoli
3cm piece of fresh ginger, peeled and finely chopped
½ fresh red chilli, deseeded and finely chopped
3 small pak choy, quartered lengthways

6. Add the ginger and chilli to the wok or pan with the pak choy (you may have to do this in batches). Fry for a few minutes until cooked, then add the broccoli back into the pan and toss.

7. Serve in bowls with the cauliflower rice, sprinkled with the coriander leaves and toasted almonds and coconut.

Tip ... A handful of green veg, such as mangetout or sugar snap peas, would be lovely in this recipe, too. Simply add to the pan with the pak choy.

JAPANESE MISO AUBERGINES

Serves 2

One of my favourite Japanese restaurants in London introduced me to miso aubergines. They're packed with flavour and are far more filling than they seem at first glance. If you fancy something to go with these, I would recommend some brown rice and stir-fried long-stemmed broccoli with garlic.

Ingredients

2 aubergines
olive oil
1 heaped tbsp brown rice miso
1 tsp coconut sugar
1 tbsp tamari
1cm piece of fresh ginger, peeled and finely chopped
2 tsp sesame seeds, to serve
1 spring onion, finely chopped, to serve

1. Preheat the oven to 180°C/350°F/gas 4.
2. Halve the aubergines lengthways, keeping the stalks intact. Scour the cut side with criss-crosses about 5mm wide. Brush lightly with olive oil and bake in the hot oven for 35 minutes.
3. Add the miso to a saucepan over a high heat with 60ml (¼ cup) water, the coconut sugar, tamari and chopped ginger and stir to combine.
4. Bring to the boil and continue to boil for 5–7 minutes until reduced and thickened.
5. When the aubergines have been baking for 35 minutes, remove from the oven and spread 1 tablespoon of the miso mixture over each half. Bake for a further 5 minutes until bubbling.
6. Remove from the oven and serve with a scattering of sesame seeds and spring onion.

Serving ideas ...

Try these with cooked wild rice tossed in lime juice and chopped coriander. Try with my Spicy Asian Tofu Salad (see page 70).

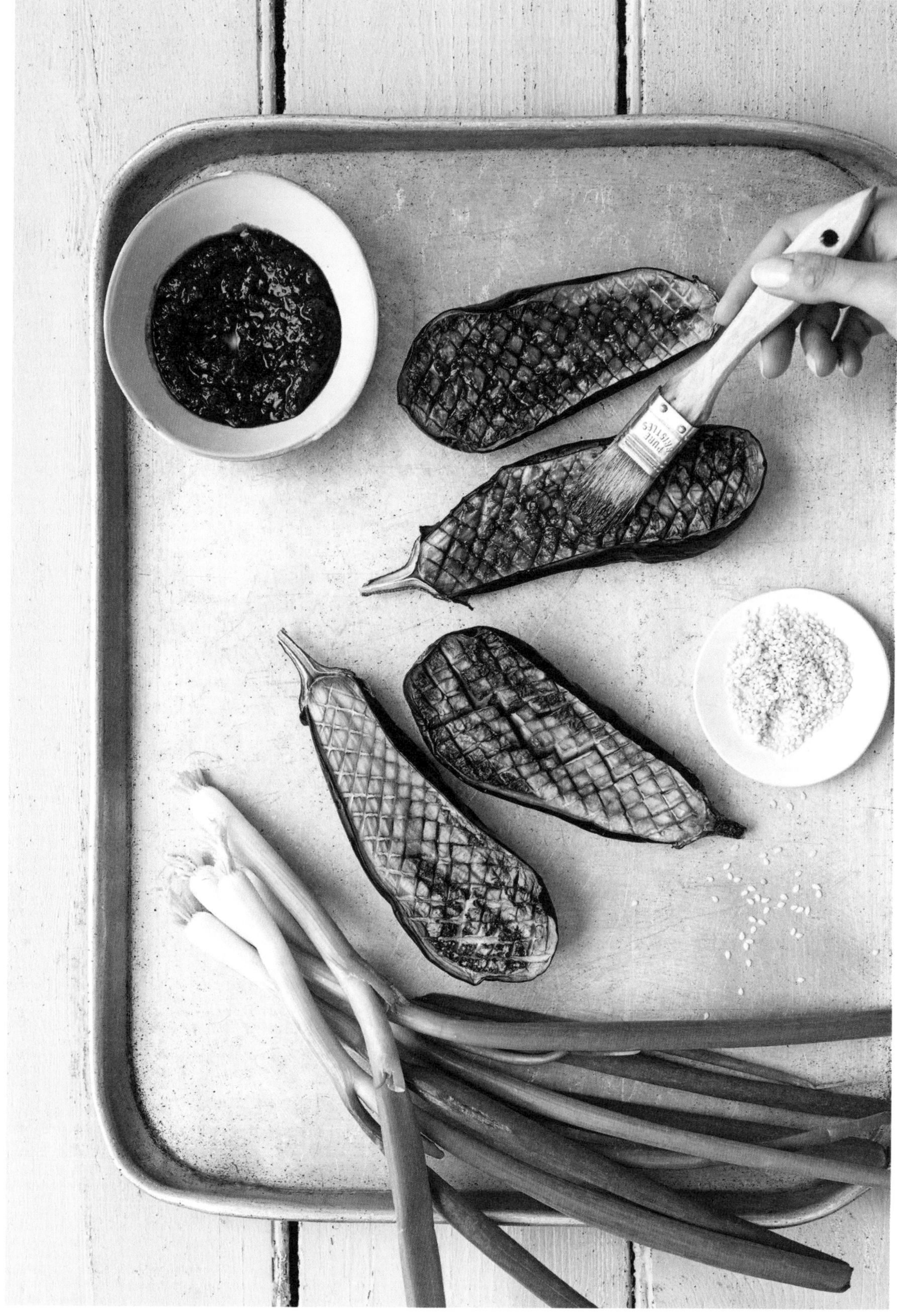

ROASTED PEPPER + ONION PESTO TART

Serves 6-8

This is a great one to make ahead. When I'm busy I often find it hard to make lunch from scratch, so I sometimes make it the night before so I know I will have something wholesome, filling and tasty ready and won't end up buying something less nutritious on the go.

Ingredients

topping
olive oil
2 red onions, peeled and each cut into 8 wedges
3 red or yellow peppers, deseeded and sliced

sweet potato tart base
1 small sweet potato (200g), peeled
150g (1 cup) spelt flour, plus extra for dusting
150g (1 cup) wholewheat flour
60ml (¼ cup) olive oil
pink Himalayan salt or sea salt

brazil nut pesto
2 garlic cloves, peeled
225g (1½ cups) unsalted raw Brazil nuts
3 large handfuls of fresh basil leaves
3 large handfuls of spinach
3 tbsp apple cider vinegar
100ml (⅜ cup) extra-virgin olive oil

1. Preheat the oven to 180°C/350°F/gas 4. Grease a 20 x 25cm shallow baking tin with olive oil.
2. Place the onion wedges and pepper slices in a roasting tray, drizzle with olive oil and roast in the hot oven for 40 minutes until cooked through and browned, tossing occasionally.
3. To make the base, chop the sweet potato into chunks and steam for 15 minutes and allow to cool.
4. Mix together the flours and a pinch of salt, then stir in the olive oil and 60ml (¼ cup) water. Mash the sweet potato and use your hands to fully combine into the mixture.
5. Flour a surface and roll out the dough to cover the base of the tin. Roll it over the tin and gently press the outer edges and corners. Use a knife to scrape away the excess from the edges. Add greaseproof paper and baking beans and bake for 15 minutes.
6. Make the pesto by adding all the pesto ingredients except 25g of the Brazil nuts to a food processor and blending for 1-2 minutes or until smooth.
7. Remove the paper and baking beans after 15 minutes, then return the tart case to the oven for a further 5 minutes.
8. Remove from the oven and generously spread the pesto on top of the base. Add the roasted veg, chop and sprinkle over the reserved Brazil nuts and bake for a further 5-7 minutes until golden and cooked through. Serve hot or cold with a lovely green salad.

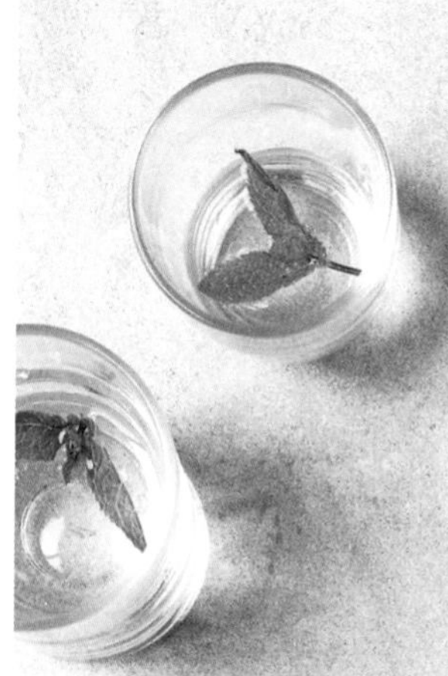

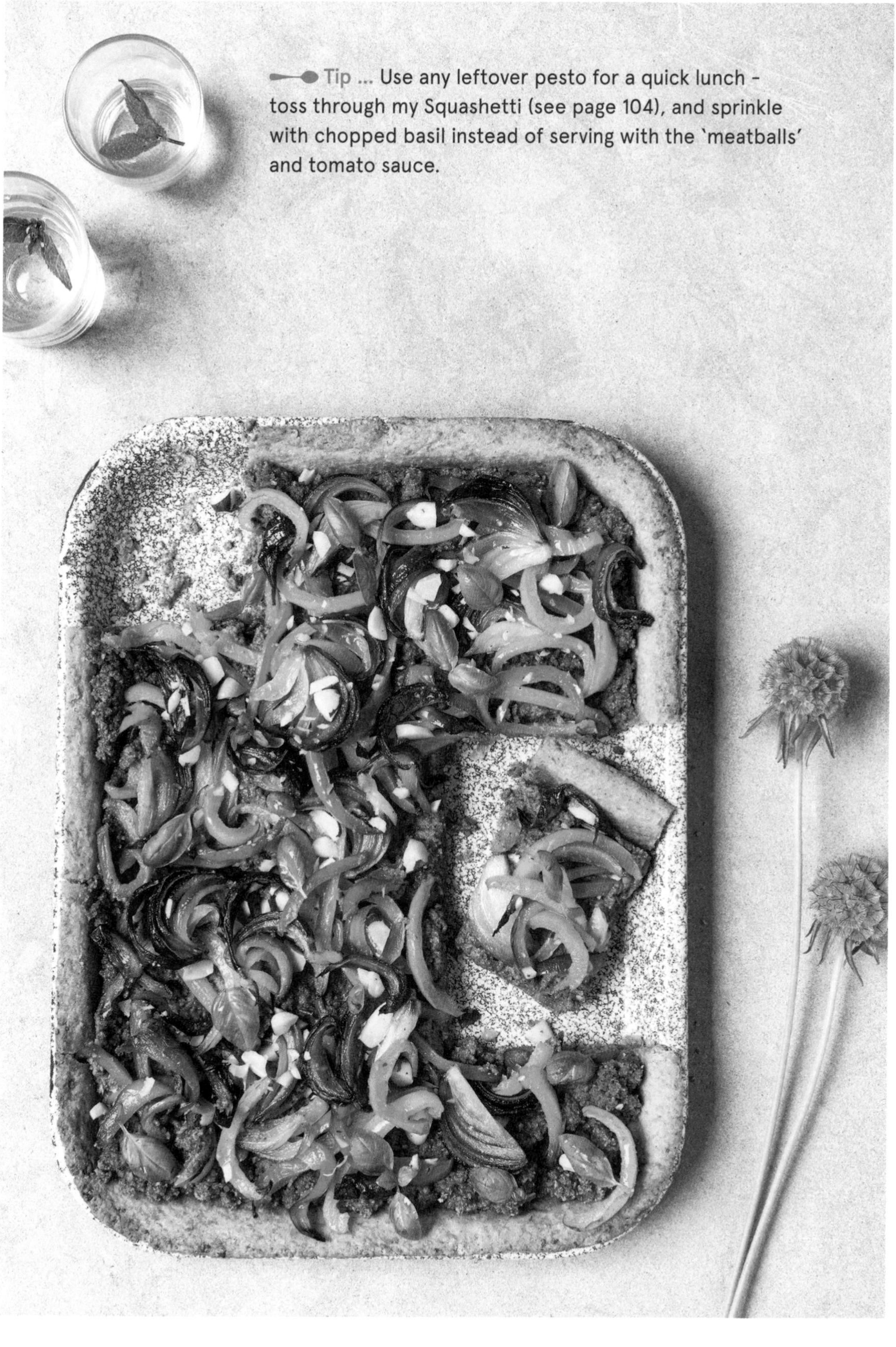

Tip ... Use any leftover pesto for a quick lunch - toss through my Squashetti (see page 104), and sprinkle with chopped basil instead of serving with the 'meatballs' and tomato sauce.

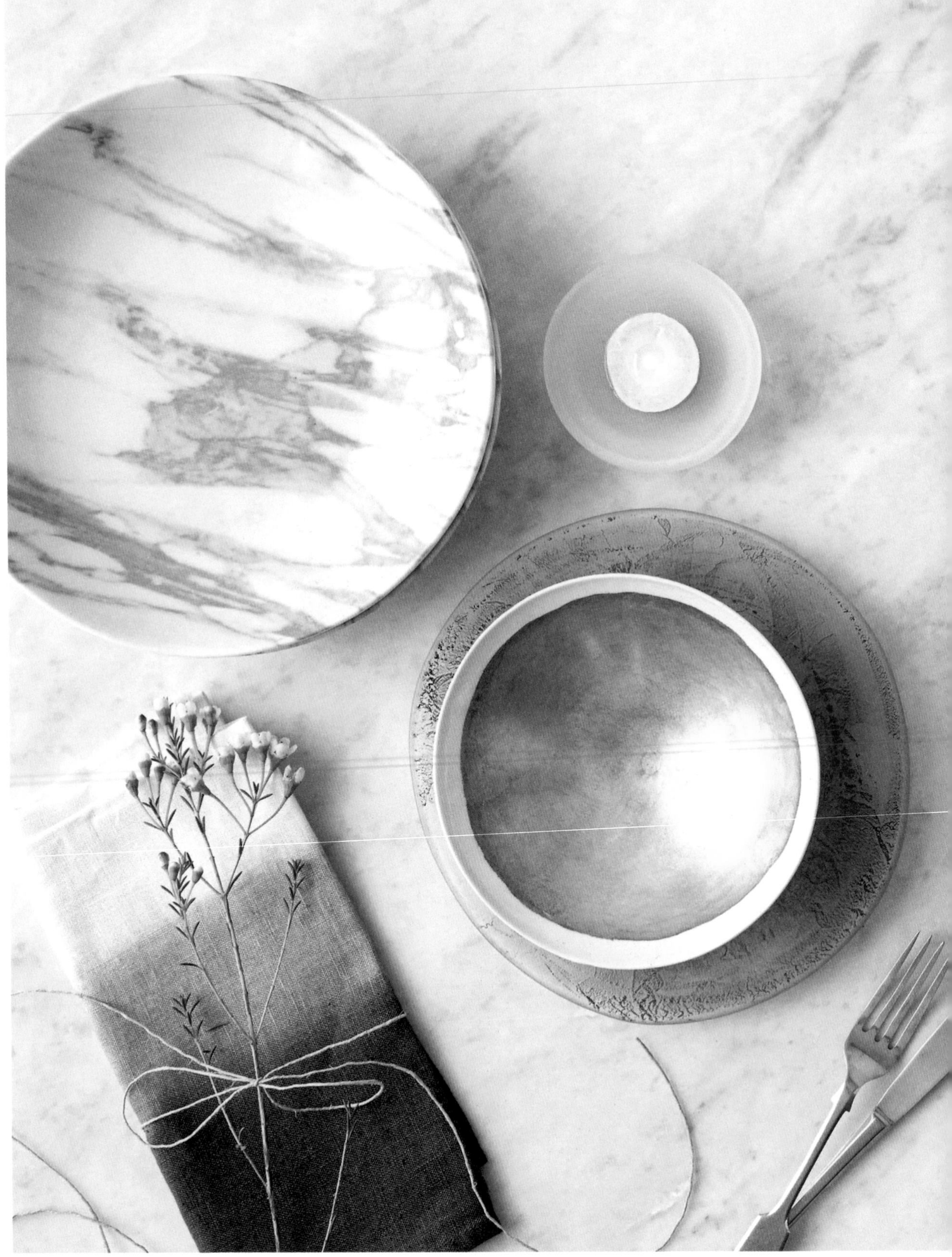

Dinner

03

MEXICAN CHILLI BOWL

Serves 2

Mexican is one of my favourite cuisines. This is a twist on the popular classic chilli con carne. I love recreating traditional home-comfort foods, all made from wholesome ingredients. I've replaced rice with quinoa, soured cream with soured coconut cream and loaded the chilli with vegetables and beans.

Ingredients

1 onion, diced
1 tsp coconut oil
2 garlic cloves, peeled and crushed
1 red pepper, deseeded and sliced into strips
6 button mushrooms, chopped
60ml (¼ cup) red wine or vegetable stock
1 tsp yeast extract
1 x 400g tin chopped tomatoes
2 tbsp tomato purée
1 x 400g tin kidney beans, drained
1 bay leaf
1 tsp ground cumin
½ tsp paprika
1 tsp dried oregano
1 tsp dried thyme
½ tsp chilli powder
150g (¾ cup) quinoa, rinsed
½ organic low-salt vegetable stock cube
pink Himalayan salt or sea salt and freshly ground black pepper

soured coconut cream

1 x 400g tin coconut milk, refrigerated
2 tbsp nutritional yeast
a squeeze of lemon juice

1. Fry the onion in the coconut oil over a medium heat for 5-7 minutes, until softened. Add the crushed garlic and continue to fry for another couple of minutes.
2. Add the pepper, mushrooms, red wine or veg stock with the yeast extract. Turn the heat down to medium-low and simmer for 5 minutes.
3. Add the chopped tomatoes, tomato purée and kidney beans with the bay leaf and remaining spices and herbs and season with a pinch of salt and black pepper.
4. Bring to the boil, then simmer over a medium-low heat for 15-20 minutes until thickened.
5. Place the quinoa in a saucepan over a medium heat. Fry off the excess water for about 30-45 seconds to help remove the earthy taste, but don't let it burn. Add 375ml (1½ cups) cold water with the stock cube and bring to the boil. Turn the heat down to low and simmer for 15 minutes until absorbed, adding more water if needed. Set aside to cool.
6. To make the soured cream, scoop out half the solid coconut cream that has risen to the top of the tin of coconut milk (this should be around 75g) and whisk with the other soured cream ingredients in a large bowl.
7. Serve the chilli with the quinoa and soured cream and dig in.

Serving ideas ...

Summer Salsa (see page 158).
Guacamole (see page 158).
Black Bean Dip (see page 163).
A small handful of coriander leaves.

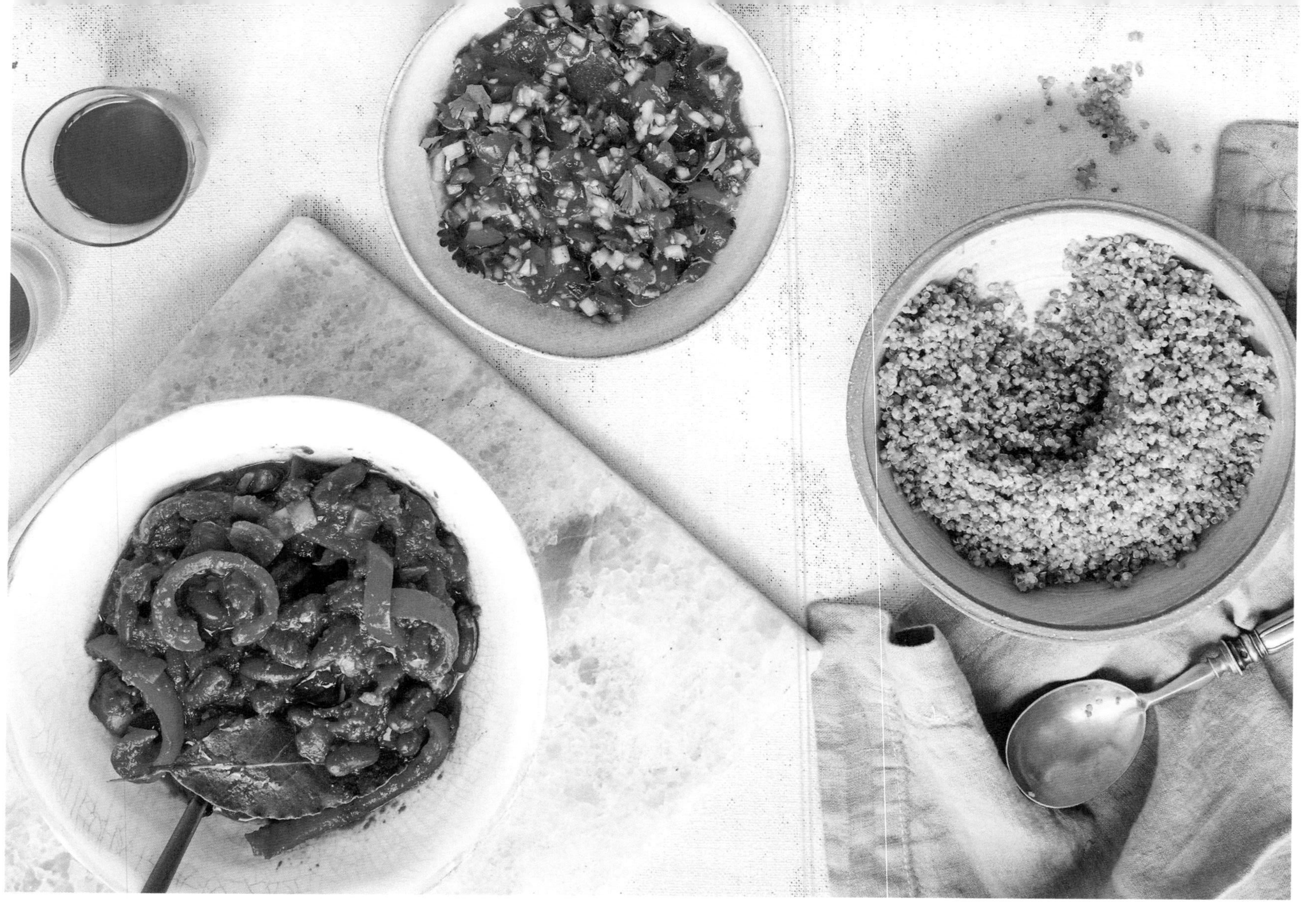

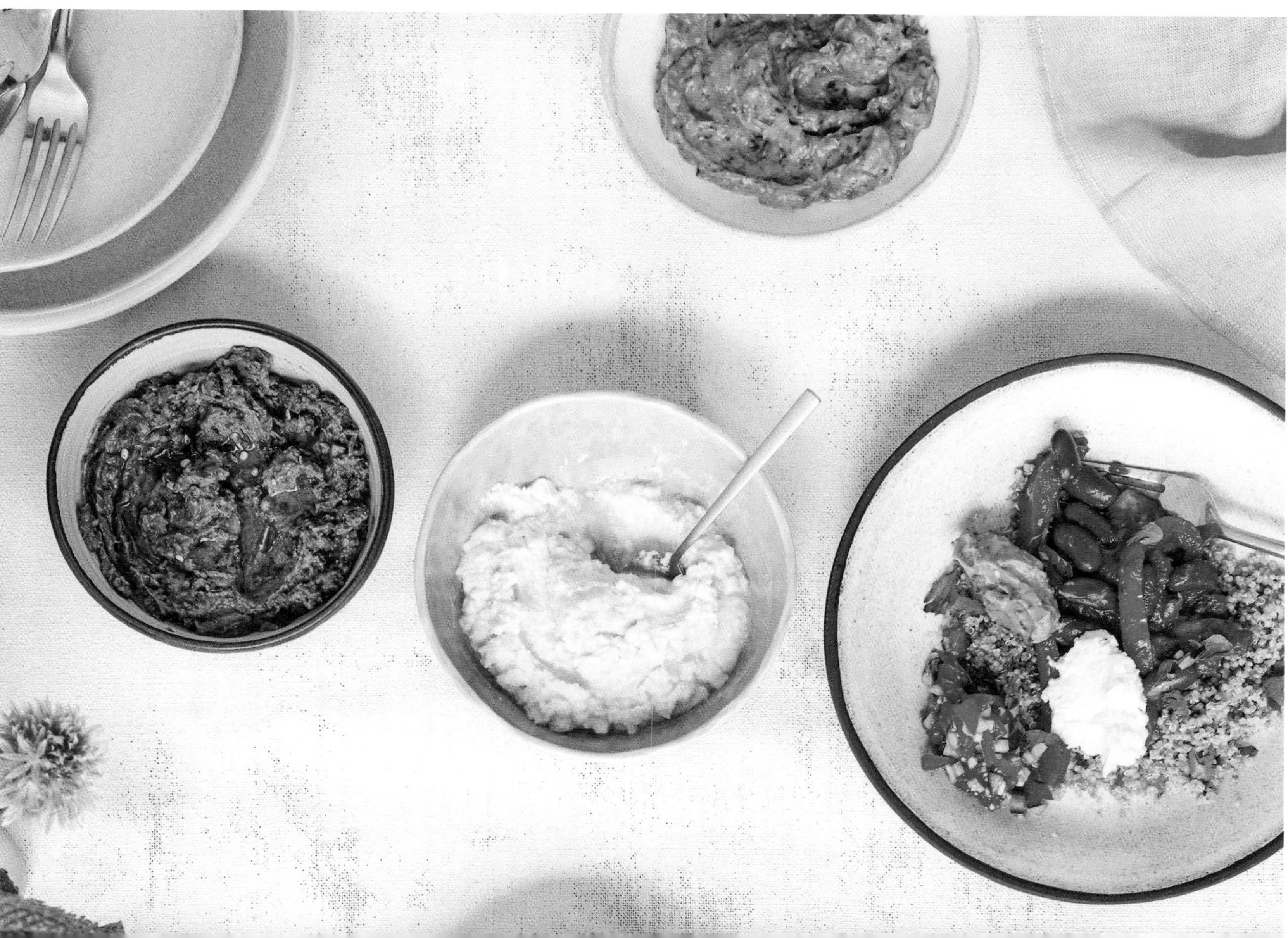

BEETROOT BURGERS

Serves 4

Veggie burgers are a common alternative at barbecues and picnics but I often find they're bland and stodgy. I've created these using beetroot for a different texture, with a hint of sweetness from apricots and mild spiciness from the cayenne pepper.

Ingredients

3 beetroots, peeled and grated
1 tsp coconut oil
1 red onion, chopped
2 garlic cloves, peeled and crushed
2½ tbsp milled flaxseed
1 x 400g tin cannellini beans, drained
4 unsulphured dried apricots
30g (¼ cup) pumpkin seeds
2 tbsp lemon juice
1 tsp dried oregano
¼ tsp cayenne pepper
1 tsp ground cumin
pink Himalayan salt or sea salt and freshly ground black pepper
8 large gem or round lettuce leaves, to serve
2 ripe beef tomatoes, sliced, to serve
2 ripe avocados, sliced, to serve
2 large radishes, sliced, to serve
wholegrain mustard, to serve

1. Preheat the oven to 190°C/375°F/gas 5.
2. Use kitchen paper to roughly dry the grated beetroot.
3. Heat the coconut oil in a frying pan and fry the onion for 5 minutes, until softened, then add the garlic, fry for a further minute, remove from the heat and set aside.
4. Mix together the flaxseed and 3 tablespoons water in a small bowl and keep to one side to thicken.
5. In a food processor, pulse the beans, apricots and pumpkin seeds a few times – you want it to be still relatively chunky. Add the lemon juice, dried oregano, cayenne pepper and cumin with a pinch of salt and black pepper and pulse again.
6. Tip into a large bowl, add the grated beetroot, flaxseed mixture and onion and mix together.
7. Take a quarter of the mixture and form a ball. Lay it on a baking sheet and gently press down to make it into a burger size. Repeat three more times.
8. Bake the burgers in the hot oven for 40 minutes, until cooked through, flipping them over halfway through.
9. Once cooked, serve in the lettuce leaves with sliced tomato, avocado, sliced radish and a little wholegrain mustard.

Serving ideas ...

Serve with my Spiced Wedges (see page 150), and my Homemade Tomato Ketchup (see page 154).

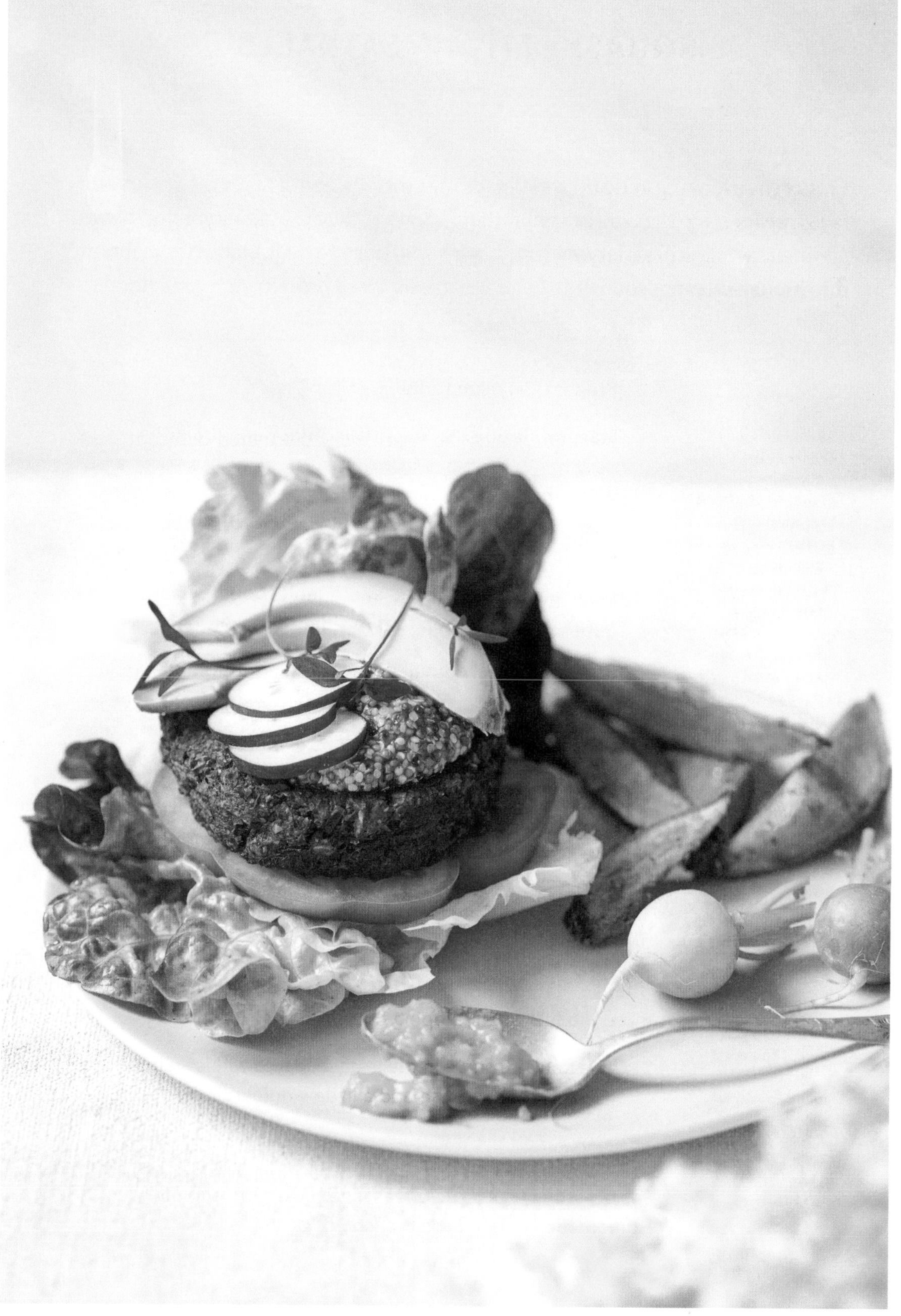

SQUASHETTI + 'MEATBALLS'

Serves 4

Rather than looking at healthy eating as missing out, think of it as altering your favourite meals so that you can enjoy them knowing they're loading your body with goodness while still satisfying your taste buds. Here pasta is made from vibrant, nutritious butternut squash and the 'meatballs' from protein-rich wholefoods.

Ingredients

'meatballs'

- 100g (½ cup) dried green lentils
- 1 onion, finely diced
- 1 teaspoon coconut oil
- 1 garlic clove, peeled and diced
- 100g (1 cup) unsalted raw walnuts
- ½ x 400g tin black beans, drained and rinsed
- 2 tbsp buckwheat flour
- 1 tsp dried oregano
- 1 tsp dried basil
- 8 unsulphured dried apricots, finely diced

- 1 x Tomato Sauce recipe, page 109
- pink Himalayan salt or sea salt and freshly ground black pepper
- a handful of fresh basil leaves, to serve
- a sprinkling of nutritional yeast (optional)

squashetti

- 2 butternut squash (approx. 1.2kg each)
- olive oil

1. Preheat the oven to 180°C/350°F/gas 4.
2. Start by making the 'meatballs'. Rinse and drain the lentils, tip into a saucepan and cover with water. Place over a medium-high heat and bring to the boil. Turn the heat down to low and simmer for 30 minutes until cooked or according to the packet instructions.
3. Fry half the onion in the coconut oil for 6–8 minutes, until softened, adding the garlic for the final minute.
4. In a food processor, pulse the walnuts a couple of times until they are in small chunks. Add the remaining meatball ingredients apart from the reserved onion and apricots, with a pinch of salt and black pepper and the cooked onion, garlic and lentils, and blend until combined. Stir in the raw diced onion and apricots.
5. Form the meatball mixture into 12 ping-pong-sized balls, place on a baking tray and bake for 30 minutes, turning halfway.
6. Peel both the butternut squashes and use a spiraliser to turn the squash into noodles. Transfer to a baking dish, drizzle with olive oil, toss to coat and bake in the hot oven for about 10 minutes, turning every couple of minutes.
7. Serve the squash spaghetti in bowls, pour over the tomato sauce, add the meatballs and serve sprinkled with fresh basil leaves and nutritional yeast, if using.

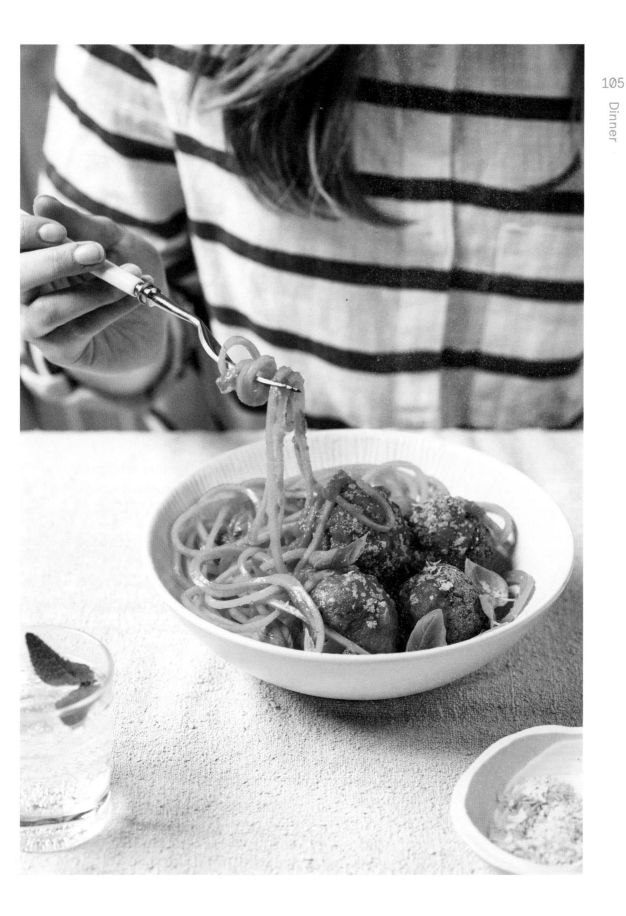

MAURITIAN MASALA WITH COCONUT CORIANDER RICE

Serves 2

When I travelled to Mauritius, I was blown away by the food. With influences from Africa, France, India and China, it was like nothing I'd ever tasted or seen before. I've adapted this traditional curry, but the fundamentals of Mauritian cooking are still at the core of this recipe.

Ingredients

200g (1 cup) brown rice, rinsed
1 tsp coconut oil
1 onion, diced
3 fresh or 6–8 dried curry leaves
2 garlic cloves, peeled and crushed
5cm piece of fresh ginger, peeled and grated
1 tbsp medium curry powder
1 tbsp turmeric
2 tsp ground cumin
200g (1 cup) butternut squash, peeled and diced
1 tbsp fresh thyme leaves, chopped
1 fresh green chilli, deseeded and diced
1 small courgette, diced
1 red pepper, deseeded and thinly sliced
2 tbsp chopped fresh coriander
2 tbsp desiccated coconut
pink Himalayan salt or sea salt
1 spring onions, trimmed and sliced, to serve

1. Tip the rice into a saucepan, cover with water and bring to the boil over a high heat. Turn the heat down to medium-low and simmer for 25 minutes or according to the packet instructions.

2. Heat the coconut oil in a frying pan over a medium heat and fry the onion with the curry leaves for about 5 minutes.

3. Add the crushed garlic and ginger and continue to fry until the onion is golden. Stir in the spices to coat the onion.

4. Add the squash with the thyme leaves, chilli and about 125ml (½ cup) water and stir well. Season with a pinch of salt and cook for a couple of minutes.

5. Now add the courgette and pepper with 250ml (1 cup) of water and simmer for about 20–25 minutes until the squash is tender. Feel free to add more water if needed, depending on your preferred consistency.

6. Once the rice is cooked, stir in most of the chopped coriander and all of the coconut.

7. Serve the curry with the rice, sprinkled with sliced spring onion and the remaining fresh coriander.

Tip … If you want to feed more people, this recipe is easy to scale up; just simmer it for longer.

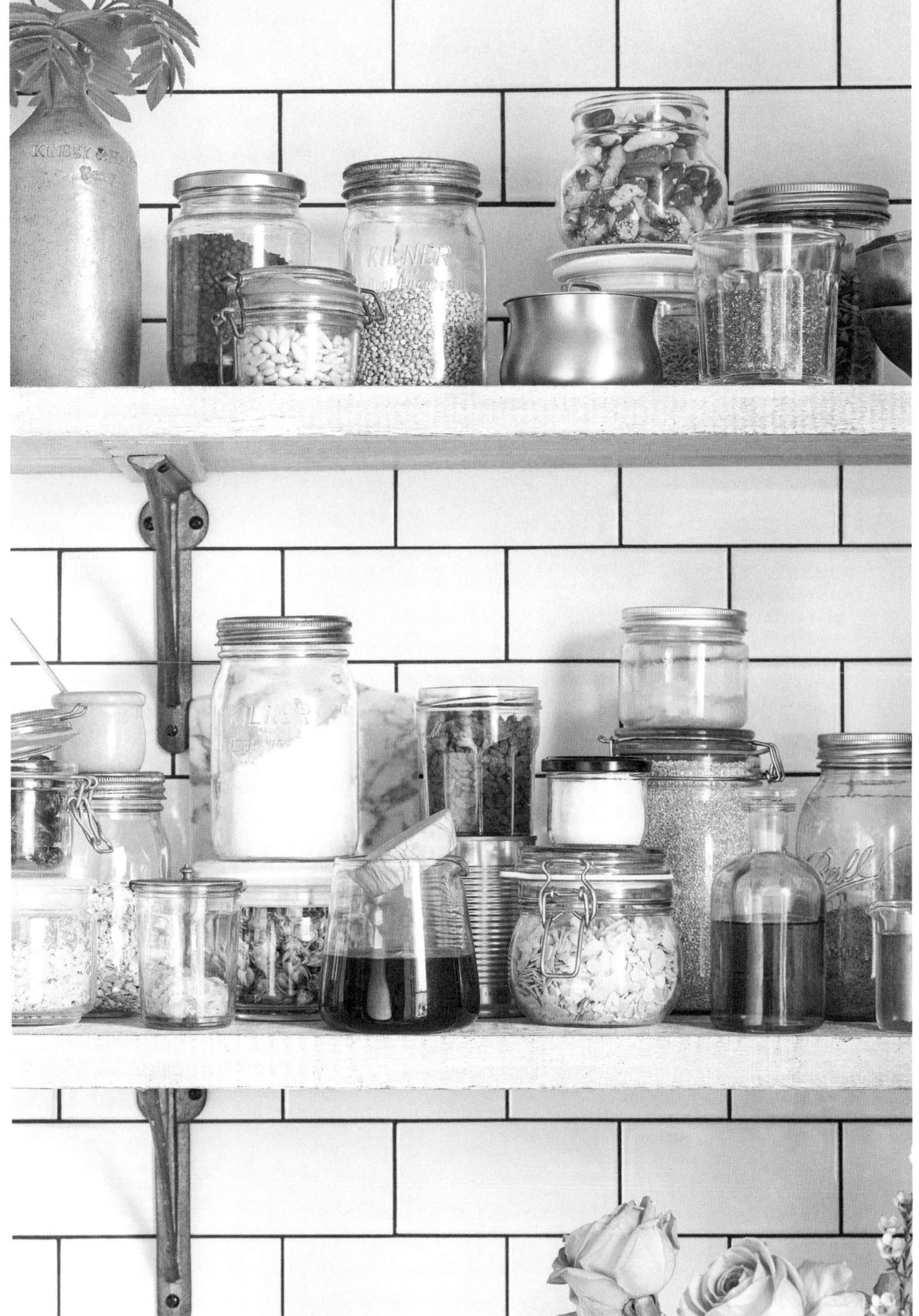
KILNER
Ball

SQUASH PIZZA – 3 WAYS

You'd think that pizza would be the first thing to go when you start eating healthily, but with this recipe you can make one that all the family will enjoy, even the biggest cheese and meat fans. I've created three different topping options, all with the same base made from butternut squash.

Ingredients

½ butternut squash (approx. 650g), peeled and chopped
2 tbsp milled flaxseed
250g (2 cups) buckwheat flour
1 tsp mixed herbs
1 tsp dried oregano
1 tbsp coconut oil, plus extra for greasing
pink Himalayan salt or sea salt and freshly ground black pepper

1. Preheat the oven to 180°C/350°F/gas 4.
2. Steam the squash for 15-20 minutes until soft and transfer to a large mixing bowl.
3. In a small bowl, mix the flaxseed with 4 tablespoons water and set aside for a few minutes to thicken up and form a gel.
4. Mash the squash until smooth, then stir in the flour with a pinch of salt and black pepper, the dried herbs and the thickened flaxseed and coconut oil. Mix together until combined. The dough will be wet but don't worry, it firms up as it bakes.
5. Grease a baking tray or a round pizza tray with a little coconut oil and smoothly spread the mixture onto it, using the back of a wooden spoon. Bake in the hot oven for 30 minutes, until lightly brown and crisp round the edges.

TOPPINGS

PESTO, TOMATO + BASIL

Serves 2

Ingredients

1 x Basil Pesto recipe (see page 159)
1 large ripe vine tomato, thinly sliced
1 tbsp pine nuts
pink Himalayan salt or sea salt and freshly ground black pepper
a handful of fresh basil leaves, to serve

1. When the butternut squash pizza base is cooked, remove from the oven and smooth over the pesto. Add the tomato slices and pine nuts and bake for another 10 minutes. Serve with the basil leaves sprinkled on top.

RED ONION, CHERRY TOMATO + ROCKET

Serves 2

Ingredients

1 x Tomato Sauce (see right)
¼ red onion, thinly sliced
¼ fresh red chilli, thinly sliced
6 ripe vine cherry tomatoes, halved
a handful of rocket leaves

1. Spread the Tomato Sauce over the baked butternut squash pizza base. Add the sliced onion, chilli and cherry tomatoes and cook for a further 10 minutes.
2. Serve sprinkled with rocket.

MUSHROOM, RED PEPPER + OLIVE

Serves 2

Ingredients

tomato sauce
½ red onion, diced
1 tsp coconut oil
4 large ripe vine tomatoes, chopped
1 garlic clove, peeled and chopped
1 tsp dried oregano
½ tsp runny honey or maple syrup
a handful of fresh basil leaves

toppings
2 mushrooms, thinly sliced
3 black olives, pitted and sliced
½ red pepper, sliced
½ tsp dried chilli flakes
½ tsp dried oregano

1. While the base is baking, make the tomato sauce. To make the tomato sauce, fry the red onion in the coconut oil over a medium heat for 5 minutes until soft.
2. Add the remaining sauce ingredients and cook over a low heat for about 15 minutes, stirring, then allow to cool. Pour into a blender and blend until smooth.
3. Spread the tomato sauce over the baked butternut squash pizza base and add the toppings. Bake for a further 10 minutes.

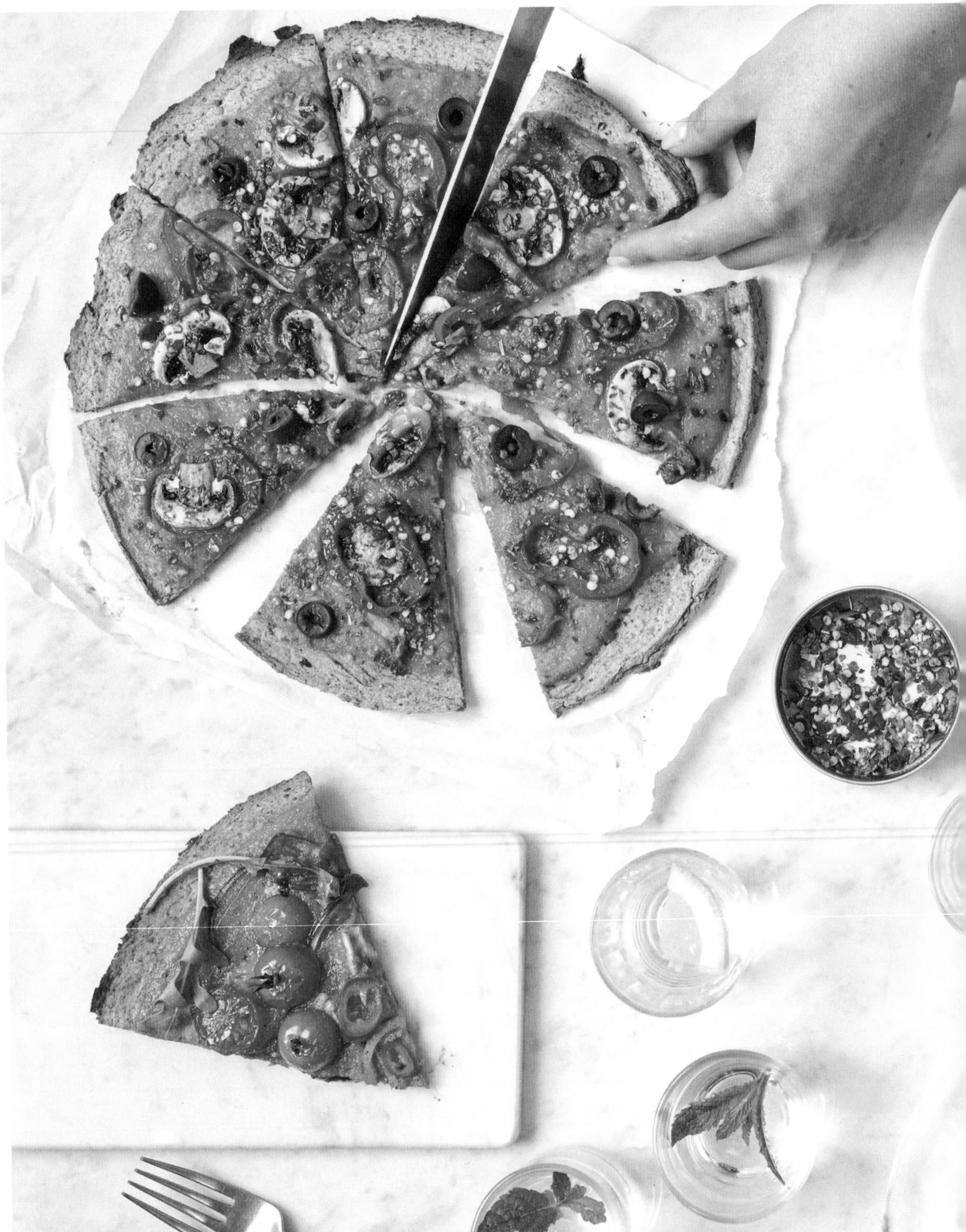

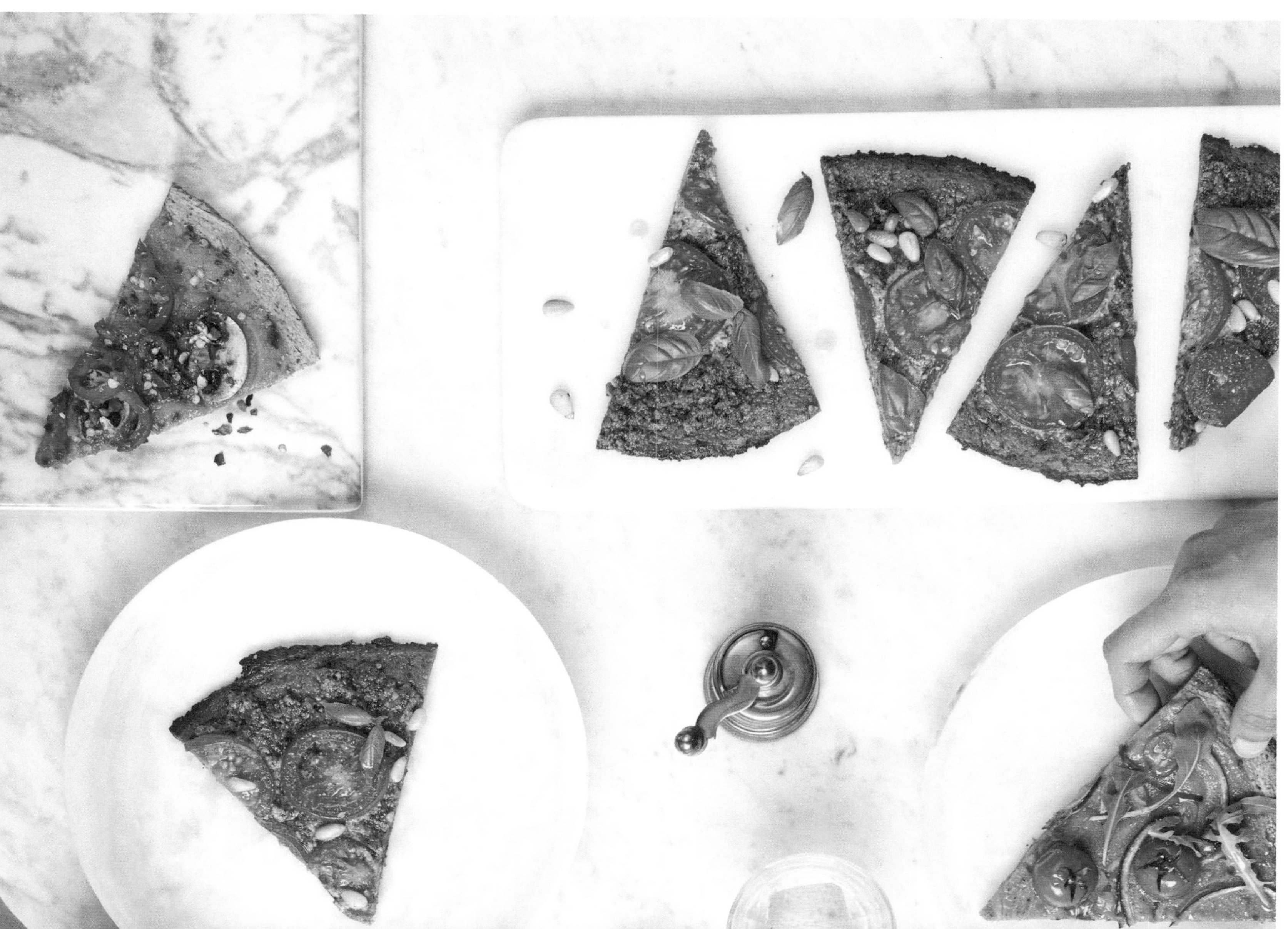

MEXICAN WILD RICE LETTUCE WRAPS

Serves 4

These are a fun way to eat healthily – place all the different components on the table so everyone can help themselves. I love Mexican food, so I wanted to make a healthier version of the popular fajita with all the flavour and colour.

Ingredients

- 2 red onions, sliced
- 2 peppers, deseeded and sliced
- 2 tbsp olive oil
- 2 large portobello mushrooms, sliced
- 4 corn on the cobs
- 200g (1 cup) wild rice, rinsed
- 1 x 400g tin chopped tomatoes
- ½ fresh red chilli, deseeded and chopped
- 1 whole large or round lettuce, to serve
- 2 ripe avocados, peeled, stoned and sliced
- pink Himalayan salt or sea salt and freshly ground black pepper
- Summer Salsa, to serve (see page 158)
- Cashew Cheese, to serve (see page 159)

spice mix

- ½ tsp ground cumin
- ½ tsp dried basil
- ¼ tsp cayenne pepper
- ½ tsp smoked paprika
- pink Himalayan salt or sea salt and freshly ground black pepper

1. Preheat the oven to 190°C/375°F/gas 5.
2. Make the spice mix by combining all the spices in a small bowl with a pinch of salt and pepper and keep to one side.
3. Place the sliced onions and peppers in a roasting tray, drizzle with the olive oil and add a pinch of salt and pepper. Roast in the hot oven for 30-35 minutes, adding the mushrooms after 10 minutes.
4. Preheat the grill to medium-high.
5. Remove the husks from the corn on the cobs. Wrap each cob in tin foil and cook under the grill for 20 minutes, turning over frequently.
6. Tip the rice into a saucepan, cover with water, bring to the boil over a medium-high heat, then turn the heat down to medium-low and cook for 25 minutes or according to the packet instructions.
7. When the rice is cooked, drain any water and add the tinned tomatoes with the spice mix and chopped chilli, return to a low heat and heat for 5 minutes until warmed through. Stir in the roasted vegetables and tip into a serving bowl.
8. Serve wrapped in large lettuce leaves, sliced avocado, Summer Salsa and Cashew Cheese with the corn on the side and dig in.

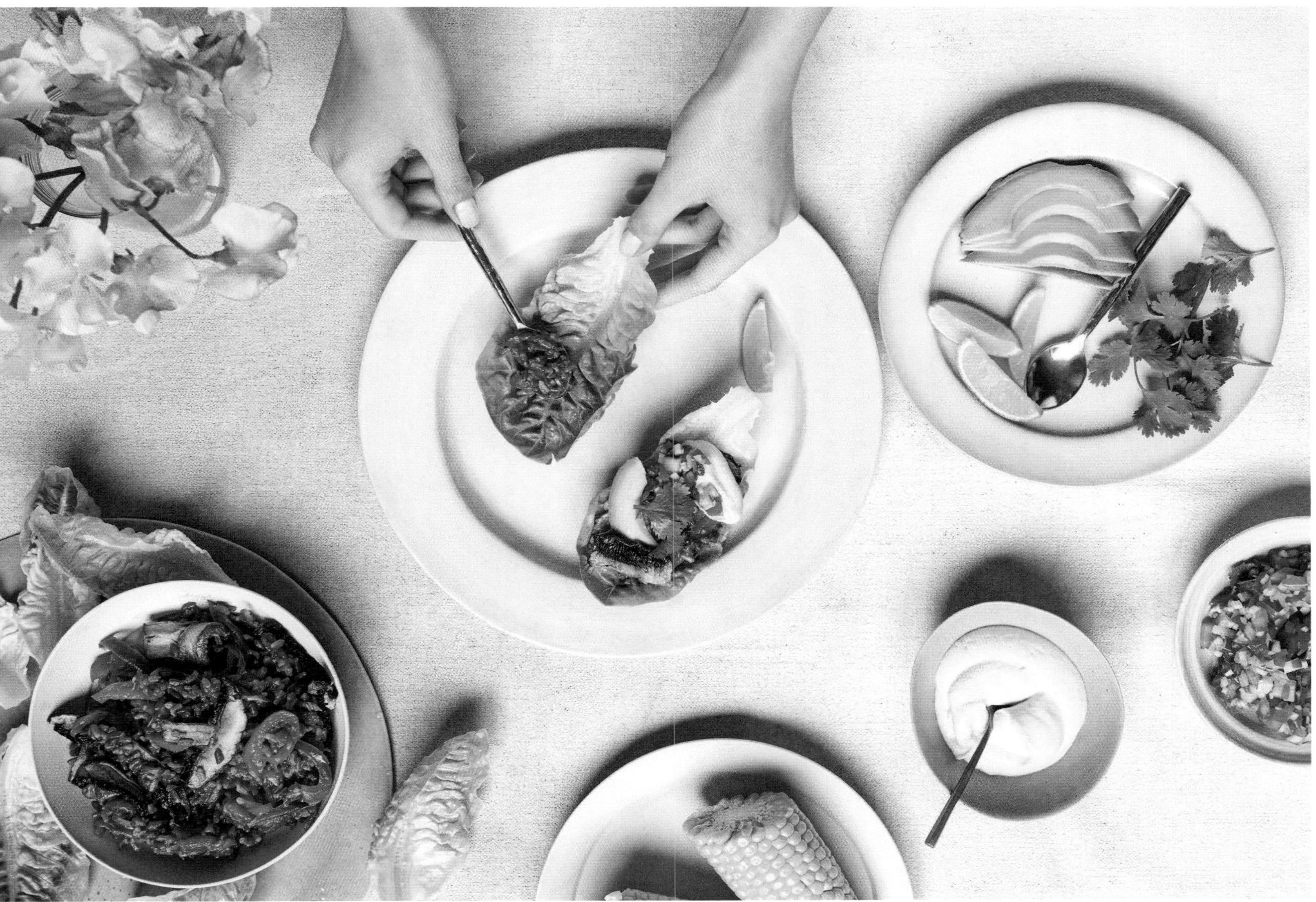

INDONESIAN KEBABS + SATAY SAUCE

Serves 4

I make these frequently during the summer to take to barbecues on the beach in Brighton. The vibrant colours and the taste of fresh vegetables with the delicious, zingy, peanut satay sauce are a perfect pairing.

Ingredients

kebabs

10 button mushrooms
2 red or yellow peppers, deseeded and chopped into 2cm chunks
1 courgette, chopped into 2cm cubes
1 red onion, chopped into 2cm cubes
12 ripe vine cherry tomatoes
1 small aubergine, chopped into 2cm cubes

satay sauce

2 tsp sesame oil
1 shallot, peeled and diced
1 garlic clove, peeled and crushed
⅓ x 400g tin coconut milk
4 tbsp smooth peanut butter
1 tbsp tamari
2 tsp runny honey
juice of ½ lime
a pinch of dried chilli flakes
a small bunch of fresh coriander, chopped, to serve
2 tbsp unsalted raw peanuts, chopped, to serve
1 lime, cut into wedges, to serve

1. Make the marinade simply by mixing all the ingredients together in a large bowl with a pinch of salt and black pepper.
2. Toss the vegetables in the bowl to coat, then cover with cling film and refrigerate for 1 hour.
3. If you are using wooden skewers, soak them in water for 20 minutes so they don't burn on cooking. Preheat the oven to 180°C/350°F/gas 4.
4. Thread the marinated vegetables onto metal or wooden skewers, alternating the veg each time.
5. Place on a baking sheet and cook in the hot oven until cooked through and nicely browned, turning once or twice.
6. Meanwhile, to make the satay sauce, heat the sesame oil in a non-stick saucepan over a medium heat. Fry the shallot for 6 minutes until softened, adding the garlic for the final minute and stirring occasionally.
7. Add the coconut milk with 60ml (¼ cup) water, the peanut butter, tamari, honey, lime juice and chilli flakes and simmer for 3–5 minutes until thickened, stirring often. If you prefer a smoother consistency, tip into a small blender or NutriBullet and whizz.
8. Serve the kebabs sprinkled with the chopped coriander, chopped peanuts and lime wedges, for squeezing over. Serve the peanut satay sauce on the side for dipping.

marinade
2 tbsp olive oil
1 tbsp lime juice
1 tbsp tamari
½ tsp ground cumin
pink Himalayan salt or sea salt and freshly ground black pepper

Serving ideas ...

I serve these with a green salad and some sweet potato wedges – or they go particularly well with my Avocado + Turmeric Salad with Quinoa (see page 77), as part of a picnic spread.

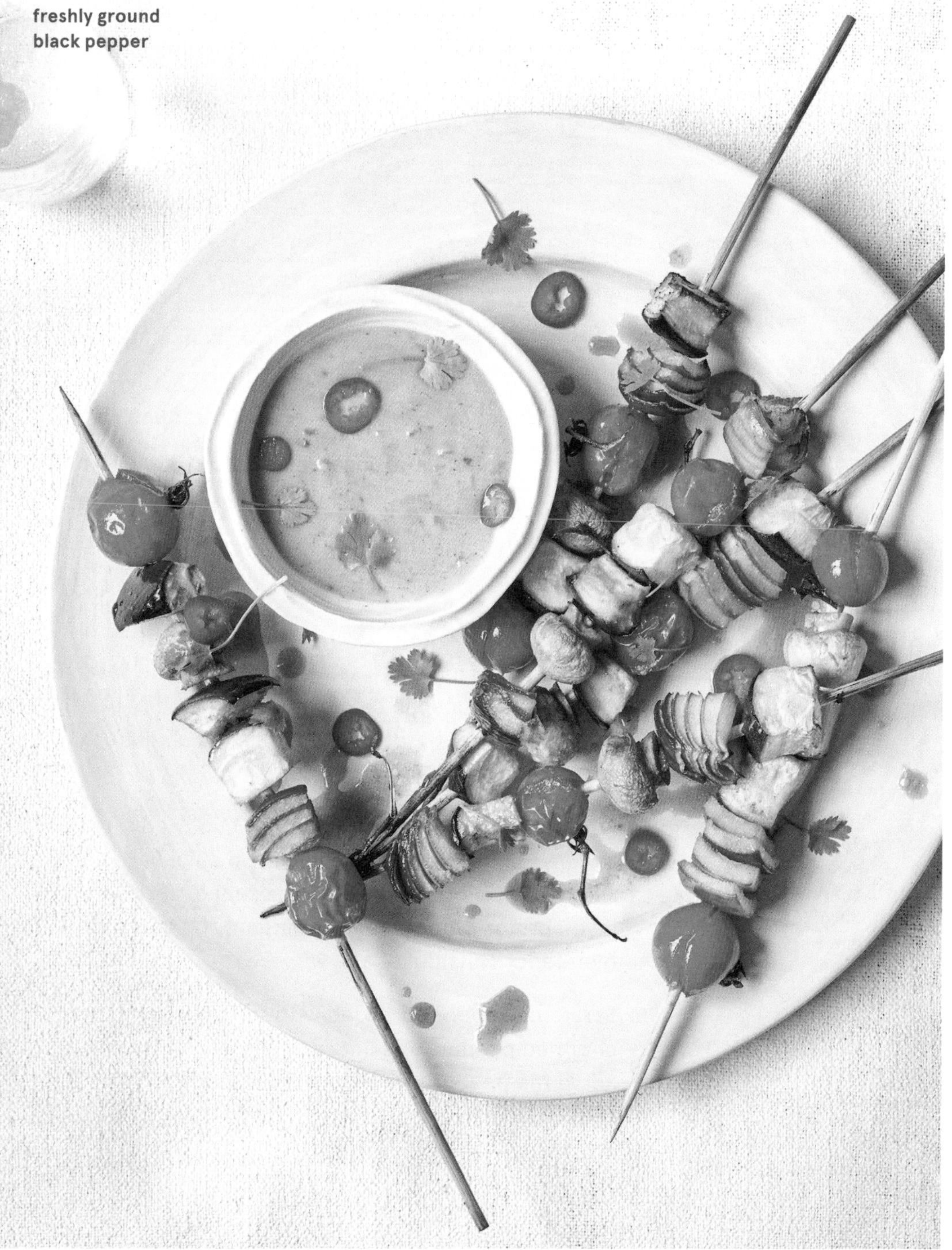

CAULIFLOWER 'STEAK' WITH CHIMICHURRI

Serves 4

You're probably thinking it's ridiculous calling this a steak, but when thickly sliced, cauliflower can be transformed into something very different to the vegetable you may be used to, it can be a great replacement for meat. The best accompaniment for this is my garlicky, herby chimichurri sauce which originates from Argentina.

Ingredients

2 large cauliflowers
1 tbsp olive oil

chimichurri sauce
2 shallots, peeled and chopped
6 garlic cloves, peeled and chopped
½–1 fresh red chilli, deseeded and chopped
1 bunch of fresh parsley, leaves chopped
1 bunch of fresh coriander, leaves chopped
125ml (½ cup) extra-virgin olive oil
4 tsp dried oregano
4 tbsp apple cider vinegar
juice of 1 lime
pink Himalayan salt or sea salt and freshly ground black pepper

1. Preheat the oven to 180°C/350°F/gas 4.
2. To make the chimichurri sauce, simply place all the ingredients in a blender and blitz to a rough paste, adding extra oil or water if needed.
3. Remove the outer leaves of the cauliflower and slice lengthways into 1cm thick slices. Try to cut at least four whole steaks from each cauliflower, enough for two each.
4. Heat the oil in a large frying pan over a high heat. Once hot, fry the cauliflower steaks for 1 minute on each side – you will need to do this in batches.
5. Transfer onto a baking tray and rub about 8 tablespoons of the chimichurri sauce over all the slices on each side. Cook in the hot oven for 25 minutes, or until cooked through, turning halfway.
6. Serve with the remaining chimichurri sauce on top.

Tip ... Grate any pieces of cauliflower that have fallen off the slices and use for Cauliflower Rice (see page 90), another time.

Serving ideas ...
Accompany this with a couple of your favourite side dishes – I always serve this with my Spiced Wedges (see page 150), and add a salad.

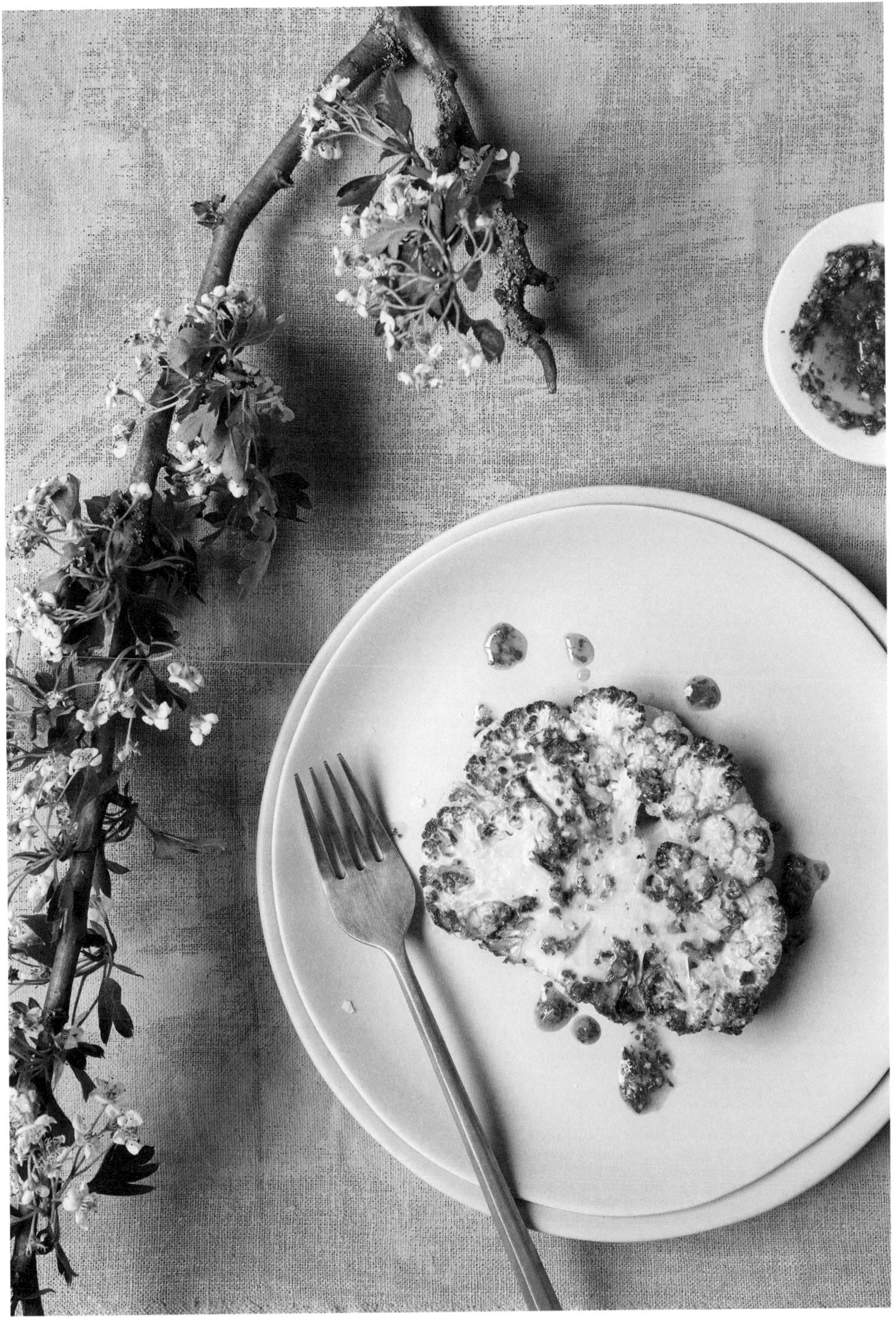

MEDITERRANEAN MEZZE

I have travelled to the Greek Islands a few times and one of my favourite things to eat out there is their traditional mezze – a platter of various Greek dishes including houmous, falafels and dolmades, so I created my own plant-based version back in rainy London.

BAKED FALAFEL

Serves 4 as part of a mezze

Ingredients

1 x 400g tin chickpeas, drained
3 garlic cloves, peeled and crushed
½ red onion, roughly chopped
1 tsp ground cumin
¼ bunch of fresh parsley, leaves picked
¼ bunch of fresh coriander, leaves picked
1 tbsp tahini
1 tbsp sesame seeds
½ tsp paprika
¼ tsp dried chilli flakes
coconut oil, for greasing
pink Himalayan salt or sea salt and freshly ground black pepper

1. Preheat the oven to 190°C/375°F/gas 5.
2. Add all the ingredients to a food processor with a pinch of salt and black pepper. Blend until the mixture holds together well, but is not entirely smooth, adding a tablespoon of water if needed.
3. Grease a baking sheet. Take heaped tablespoons of the mixture and use your hands to form them into balls. Place on the baking sheet, pat down to slightly flatten them and bake for 30 minutes, turning halfway.

SPRING GREEN DOLMADES

Serves 4 as part of a mezze

Ingredients

100g (½ cup) brown rice, rinsed
1 tsp olive oil
½ onion, finely diced
2 garlic cloves, peeled and crushed
¼ red pepper, deseeded and finely diced
a couple of sprigs each of fresh parsley, mint and dill, finely chopped
4 unsulphured dried apricots, finely chopped
juice of 1 lemon
1 tbsp tahini
13 spring green leaves
pink Himalayan salt or sea salt and freshly ground black pepper
extra-virgin olive oil, to serve

1. Tip the rice into a saucepan, cover with water and bring to the boil over a high heat. Turn the heat down to medium-low and simmer for 25 minutes or according to the packet instructions.
2. Meanwhile, heat the olive oil in a frying pan over a medium-high heat and fry the onion for 5-7 minutes until softened. Add the garlic and fry for a further minute. Add the finely diced pepper and cook for 7-10 minutes, stirring occasionally, then remove from the heat and keep to one side.

3. Once the rice is cooked, stir in the pepper and onion mixture, herbs, apricots, lemon juice and tahini. Season with salt and pepper and keep to one side.

4. Trim the thick stems off the spring green leaves and cut a triangle shape at the base of the stem where it is thickest, to remove it – this will make them easier to roll.

5. Place a saucepan of boiling water over a high heat, set a lidded steamer basket on top and steam 10 of the leaves, one at a time, for about 45 seconds each until softened – you can do this as you wrap them rather than waiting for all of them to be done.

6. Take one steamed leaf and, with the vein side up, add a tablespoon of the rice mixture to the centre. Roll over once, pull in each side and roll until you have a neat parcel like a tortilla wrap. Repeat with the remaining 9 leaves.

7. Line the steamer basket with the 3 raw leaves – this will prevent the dolmades sticking to the bottom. Place all the dolmades in the steamer on top of the leaves and steam for 15 minutes.

8. Allow to cool and refrigerate for at least an hour. These taste even better after being in the fridge overnight! When ready to serve, drizzle with a little bit of extra-virgin olive oil.

Tip ... Make this a full mezze by serving with a few other dishes such as my classic Houmous (see page 162) and My Greek Island Salad (see page 69).

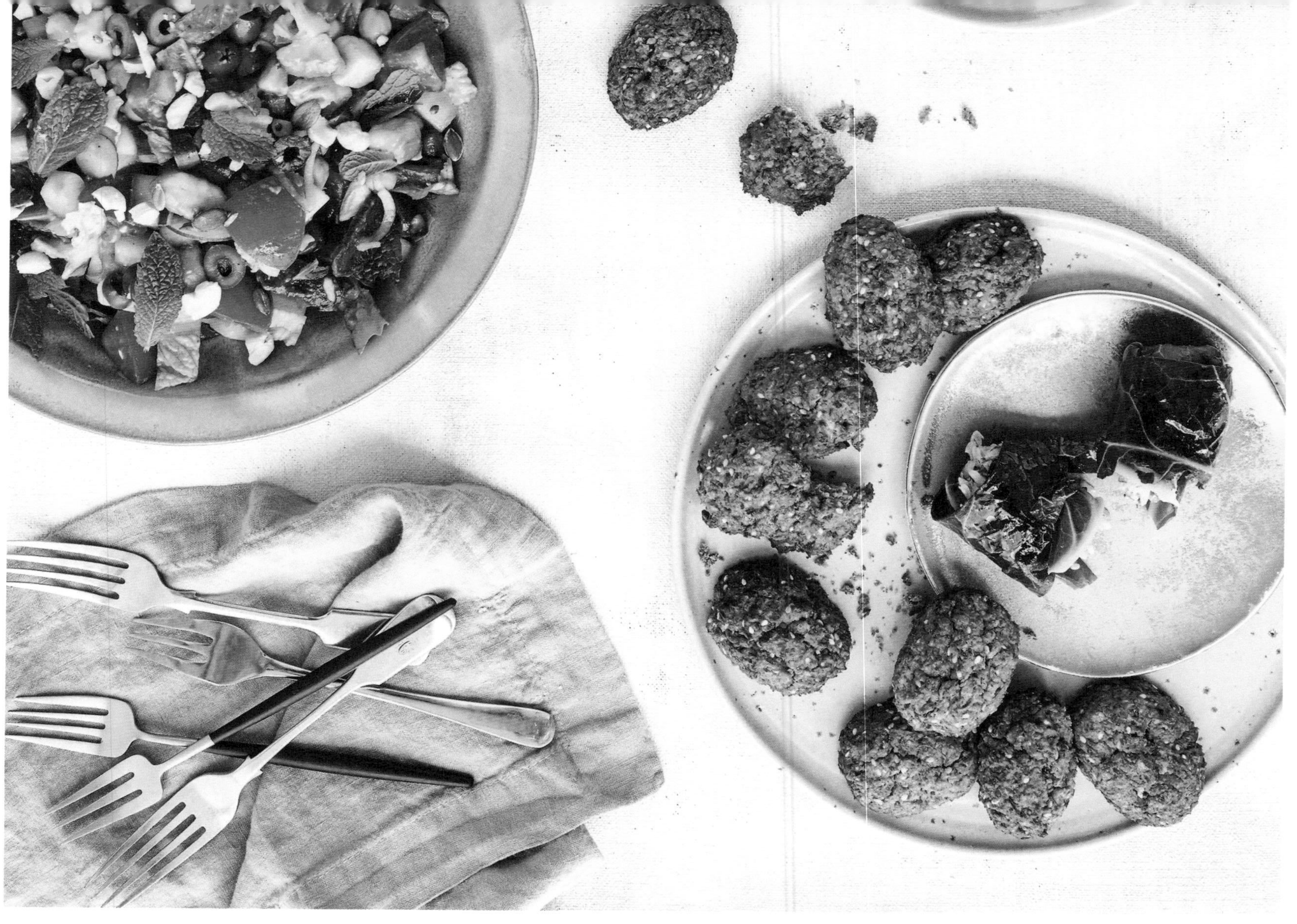

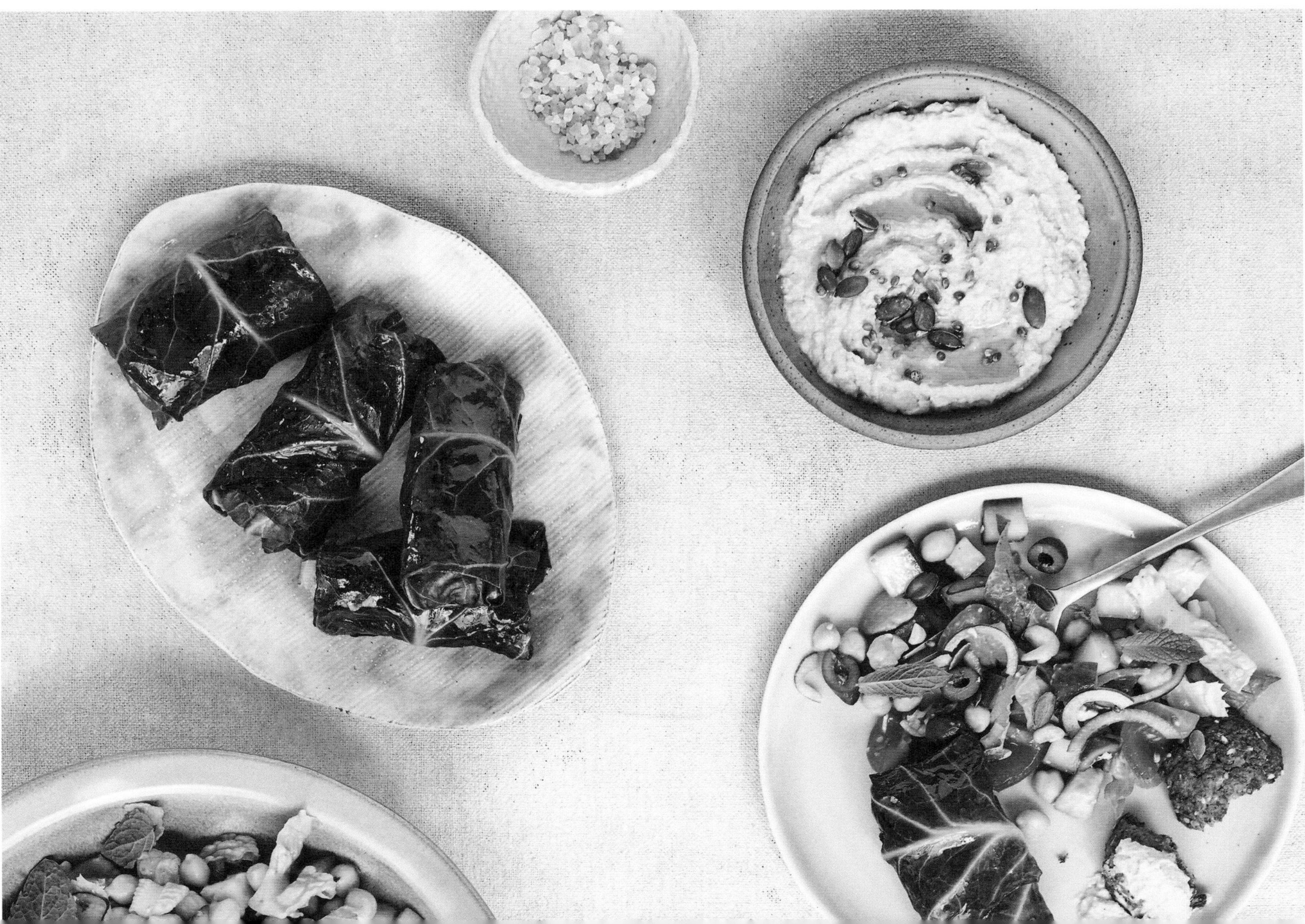

VEGETABLE LAKSA

Serves 2

I first tried laksa in Indonesia and have since had it again in Singapore, although it originates from China. Traditionally, not many vegetables are added to this dish, which consists of a curry soup and noodles, but of course I've loaded it up with various fresh vegetables. It's a perfect midweek meal.

Ingredients

paste

½ fresh red chilli, deseeded and sliced
2 garlic cloves, peeled and chopped
2–3cm piece of fresh ginger, peeled and chopped
2 shallots, peeled and chopped
juice of ½ lemon
2 tbsp tamari
a pinch of ground cloves
1 tsp coconut sugar
1 tsp turmeric

laksa

1 onion, diced
1 tsp coconut oil
1 red pepper, deseeded and sliced
8 baby corns, halved lengthways
about 20 sugar snaps
½ x 400g tin coconut milk
100g brown rice udon or buckwheat noodles
a large handful of fresh coriander leaves
2 small handfuls of beansprouts, to serve
½ spring onion, sliced, to serve
2 lime wedges, to serve

1. Start by making the laksa paste. Keep aside a few slices of chilli for garnishing at the end, then blend all the ingredients for the paste in a blender until smooth (if you have a NutriBullet, I find the milling blade works well for this). Set aside.

2. Fry the onion in the coconut oil for 5 minutes over a medium heat, then add the laksa paste to the pan and stir well.

3. Turn the heat up slightly, add the remaining vegetables and fry for a further 3–5 minutes, stirring occasionally.

4. Pour in 500ml (2 cups) water with the coconut milk and bring to a boil. Add the noodles and simmer for 7 minutes or until the noodles are cooked.

5. Stir in half the coriander and serve in bowls and sprinkle with the beansprouts, remaining coriander, spring onion and chilli slices on top with a wedge of lime each for squeezing over.

Tip ... Use the leftover coconut milk in another recipe – try my Warming Squash Soup (see page 80).

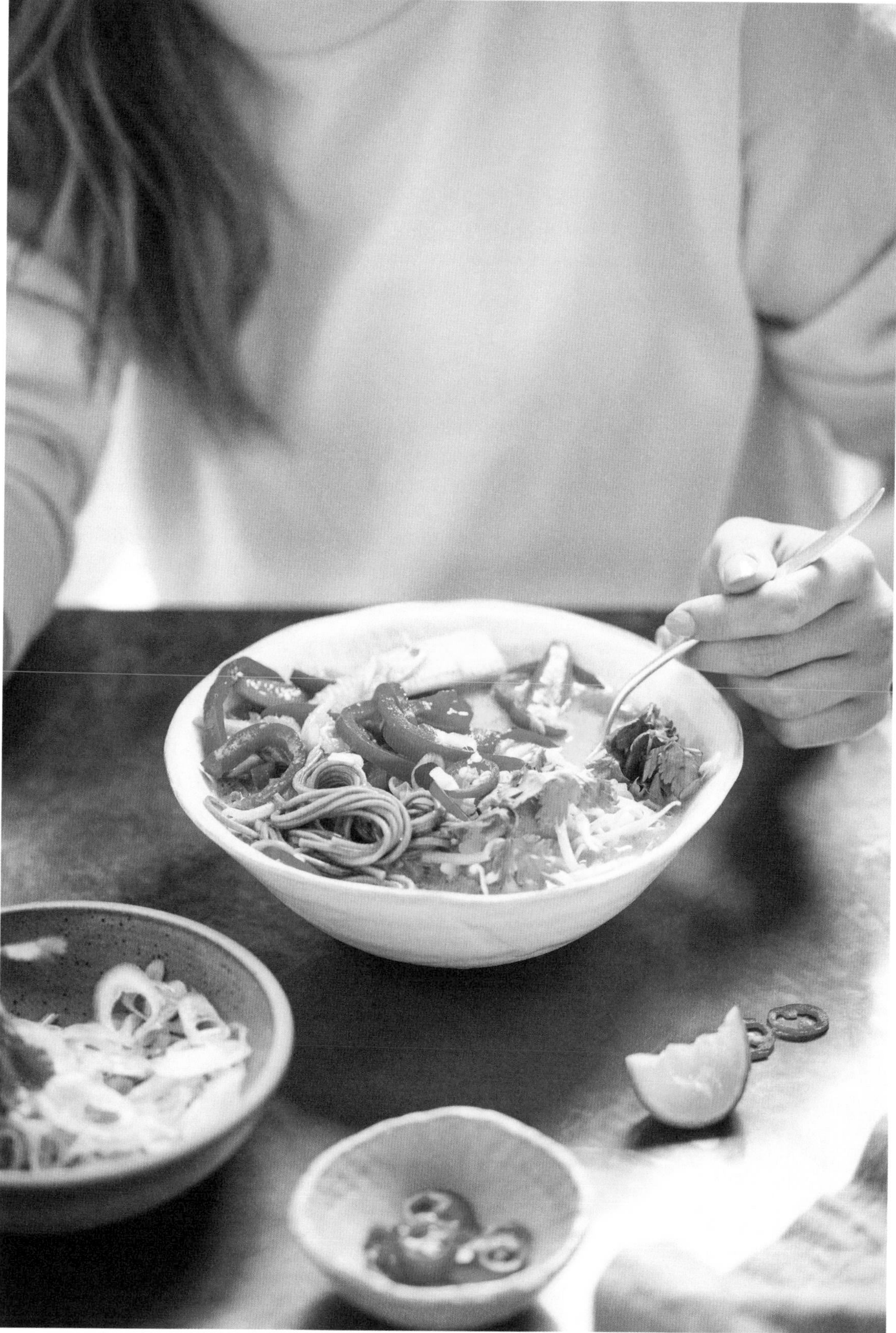

MUSHROOM MISO HOT POT

Serves 4

A regular appearance on menus at Japanese restaurants is a hot pot of rice with a delicious variety of vegetables. Because I love this dish so much I wanted to create a similar one that's easy to make at home with fresh and wholesome ingredients.

Ingredients

300g (1½ cups) brown short-grain rice
150g (1½ cups) mixed mushrooms, such as shiitake, oyster, enokitake, roughly chopped
1 leek, trimmed, sliced and rinsed
1 tbsp miso paste
1 fresh red chilli, deseeded and finely sliced
1 tbsp tamari
1 tsp coconut sugar
½ x 400g packet firm tofu, cut into small cubes
1 tsp coconut oil
a handful of enokitake mushrooms, to serve
1 spring onion, trimmed and sliced, to serve

mushroom stock

5cm piece of fresh ginger, peeled and chopped
2 garlic cloves, peeled
5 chestnut mushrooms, sliced
pink Himalayan salt or sea salt and freshly ground black pepper

1. Make the mushroom stock by bringing 1 litre (4 cups) water to the boil with the ginger, garlic, mushrooms and a pinch of salt and black pepper, then simmer for 15 minutes.
2. Add the rice, bring to the boil, stir in the mushrooms and leek and simmer for 25 minutes, until cooked, adding more boiling water if needed. Halfway through, stir in the miso paste, chilli, tamari and coconut sugar.
3. While the rice is cooking, put the tofu on a chopping board, place another chopping board on top and place a heavy pan or plate on top to press the tofu down to remove excess water. Leave for about 20 minutes.
4. Once the tofu has been weighed down for 20 minutes, drain any liquid, pat the tofu dry with kitchen paper and cut into cubes.
5. Fry the tofu in the coconut oil in a frying pan over a medium heat for 8-10 minutes until golden.
6. Once the rice is cooked, stir the tofu into the rice and serve in bowls, with the raw enokitake mushrooms and sliced spring onions on top.

Tip ... Use the extra tofu in my Spicy Asian Tofu Salad (see page 70), or Tofu Scramble (see page 62).

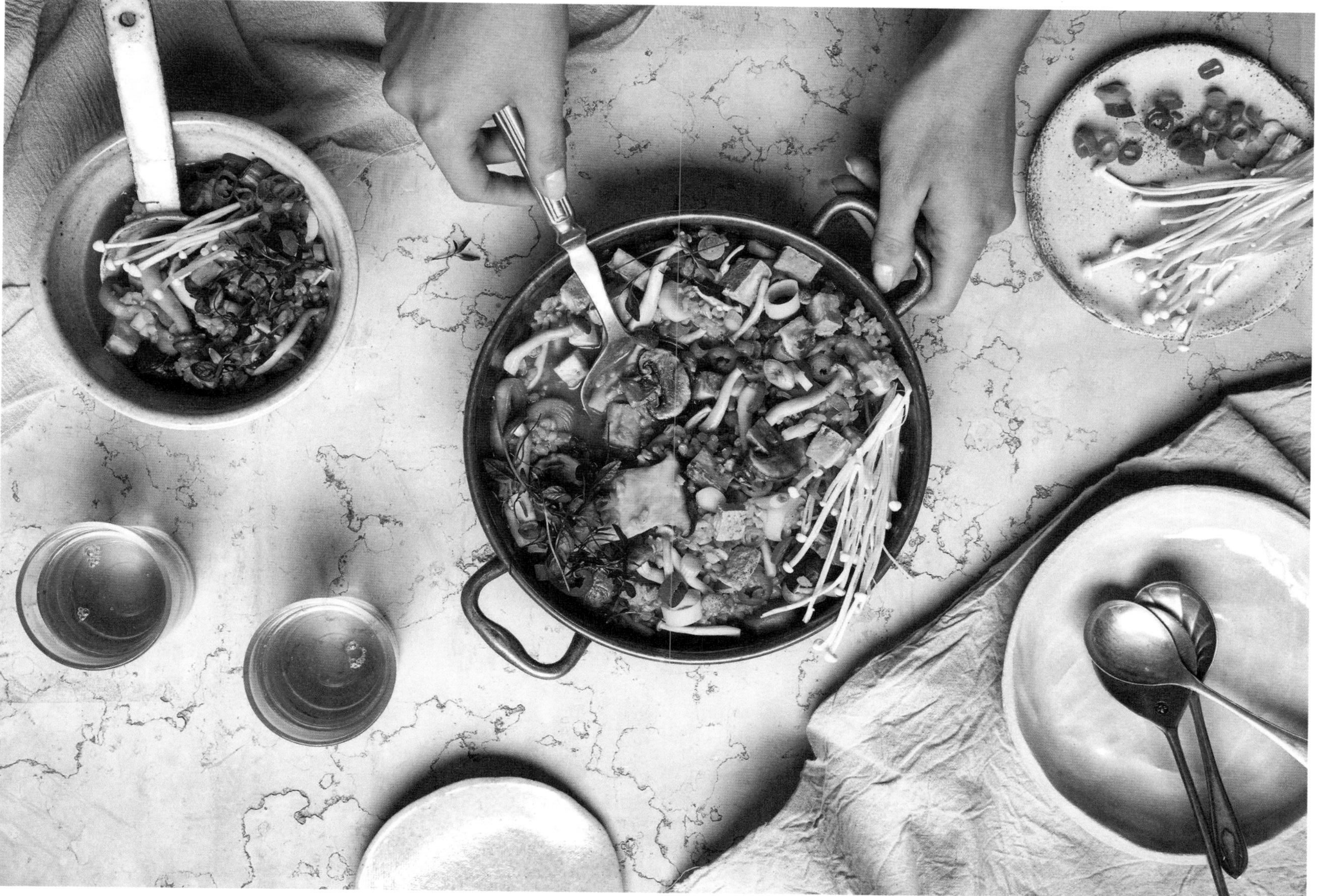

INDIAN DAHL

Serves 2

Indian food is one of my favourite cuisines because I love anything spicy. This wonderful dahl recipe is so easy to make using ingredients that you probably already have in your cupboards. It's incredibly good for you, too, high in protein and with all the wonderful natural benefits from the spices.

Ingredients

- 250g (1 cup) dried red lentils, rinsed
- 2 tsp cumin seeds
- 1 tsp mustard seeds
- 1 tsp coriander seeds
- 1 onion, peeled and diced
- 7cm piece of fresh ginger, peeled and grated
- 3 garlic cloves, peeled and crushed
- 1 tbsp coconut oil
- ½ bunch of fresh coriander, leaves picked and stalks finely chopped
- 1 tsp turmeric
- ½ tsp chilli powder
- pink Himalayan salt or sea salt
- 4 ripe vine tomatoes, chopped

1. Soak the lentils in about 750ml (3 cups) water for at least 1 hour or ideally overnight.
2. Drain the lentils and cook them in 750ml (3 cups) water. Bring to the boil, then simmer over a low heat for 15 minutes, until thickened and all the water has been absorbed.
3. Fry the cumin, mustard and coriander seeds in a dry frying pan over a medium heat for a few seconds. Remove from the heat, tip into a pestle and mortar, lightly crush, then return to the pan.
4. Grind the onion, ginger, and garlic into a paste using a pestle and mortar or a food processor.
5. Return the pan to a medium heat. Add the coconut oil with the coriander stalks, turmeric, chilli powder, a pinch of salt and the onion, ginger and garlic paste and fry for about 2 minutes.
6. Stir in the tomatoes and cook for a further 10-15 minutes, until the tomatoes have softened, then stir through the cooked lentils and sprinkle over the coriander.

Tip ... These two Indian dishes make delicious and easy midweek mains. They taste even better the next day, so save a portion for lunch. Or you can cook both dishes and serve them together for a curry night for 4.

FRIDAY NIGHT CURRY

Serves 2

At home, Friday night is curry night. One of my favourite things to eat is a curry, but they are often very high in sodium and unhealthy fats, so I decided to create my own with all the flavours but with more goodness. I've served this with wild rice and chickpeas for the high fibre content, and the chickpeas also give a protein punch.

Ingredients

190g (1 cup) wild rice, rinsed
1 tsp coconut oil
1 onion, finely diced
2 garlic cloves, peeled and crushed
5cm piece of fresh ginger, peeled and grated
1 fresh red chilli, deseeded and finely chopped
1 red pepper, deseeded and diced
1 x 400g tin chickpeas, drained
1 x 400g tin chopped tomatoes
a large handful of spinach
pink Himalayan salt or sea salt and freshly ground black pepper
¼ bunch of fresh coriander, leaves picked, to serve
1 lemon, cut into wedges, to serve

spice mix

½ tsp chilli powder
½ tsp garam masala
1 tsp ground cumin
1 tsp turmeric
1 tsp ground coriander

1. Cook the rice according to the packet instructions.
2. Mix the spice mix ingredients together in a small bowl.
3. Heat the coconut oil in a medium saucepan over a medium heat and fry the diced onion for 5–7 minutes.
4. Add the garlic, ginger and fresh red chilli, to taste, to the pan and fry for a minute or two.
5. Now add the spice mix, bit by bit, with the diced pepper, chickpeas and chopped tomatoes. Use the empty tomato tin to half fill with water and add to the pan. Add more spice mix until it is as spiced as you like it. I tend to add all of it.
6. Place a lid on the saucepan and simmer for 10 minutes, then remove the lid and simmer for a further 10 minutes.
7. Once cooked, stir in the spinach, season to taste with salt and pepper and serve with the rice, sprinkled with the coriander leaves and with a wedge of lemon on the side.

SHEPHERD'S PIE

Serves 4

This is my ultimate comfort food, perfect for a cosy winter night in. To get the 'meaty' consistency here I've combined mushrooms, walnuts and lentils which provide a wonderful taste and texture, topped with delicious parsnips and potato.

Ingredients

100g (½ cup) dried green lentils
1 onion, chopped
olive oil
1 garlic clove, peeled and chopped
2 carrots, peeled and diced
200g (2 cups) chestnut mushrooms, diced
100g (1 cup) unsalted raw walnuts, finely chopped
150g (1 cup) peas
125ml (½ cup) red wine (optional)
½ organic low-salt vegetable stock cube
1 tsp yeast extract
1 x 400g tin chopped tomatoes
1 tsp mixed dried herbs

topping

4 parsnips, peeled and chopped
2 medium potatoes, peeled and chopped
250ml (1 cup) unsweetened almond milk
a couple of sprigs of fresh thyme, leaves picked
pink Himalayan salt or sea salt and freshly ground black pepper

1. Preheat the oven to 200°C/400°F/gas 6. Start by cooking the lentils according to the packet instructions.
2. While the lentils are cooking, cook the parsnips and potatoes for the topping. Place both in a saucepan, cover with cold water, bring to the boil and cook for 20 minutes or until soft.
3. Meanwhile, set a large saucepan over a medium-high heat and fry the onion in a little olive oil for 5 minutes until softened, stirring regularly.
4. Add the garlic, carrots and mushrooms to the pan. Fry for a couple more minutes, then remove from the heat and set aside.
5. Once the lentils are cooked, drain and add them to the saucepan along with the walnuts and peas.
6. Pour 125ml (½ cup) boiling water into a jug, add the red wine or replace with extra water (if not using), the stock cube and yeast extract and stir to dissolve.
7. Pour into the pan along with the tinned tomatoes and dried herbs and stir. Bring to the boil, then turn the heat down to medium-low and simmer for about 15 minutes.
8. When the parsnips and potatoes are cooked, drain and mash with the almond milk and salt and black pepper until smooth.
9. Transfer the cooked vegetables and lentils to a baking dish and evenly spoon over the parsnip and potato mash, right to the edges of the dish, using a fork to fluff up the mash.
10. Toss the thyme in olive oil, sprinkle over the mash and bake in the hot oven for 30 minutes or until golden.

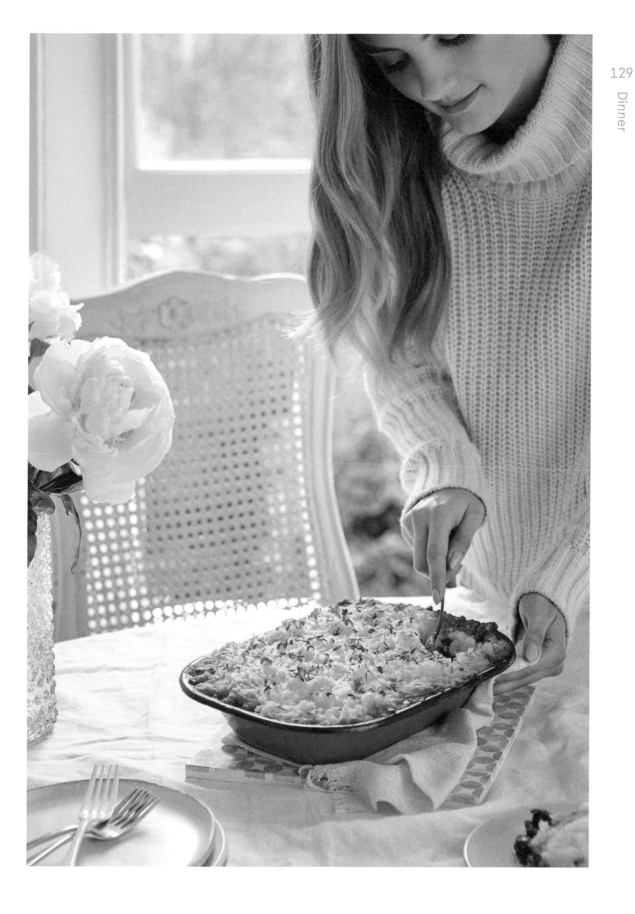

ITALIAN STUFFED PEPPERS

Serves 4

When I went to one of the best Italian restaurants (the Four Seasons, in Mauritius of all places), I ate a traditional stuffed pepper. It wasn't the healthiest but I loved it so much I decided to make my own version, with brown rice, an abundance of vegetables and a slight crunch from pine nuts.

Ingredients

- 200g (1 cup) brown rice
- 4 large red peppers
- 2 tbsp olive oil
- 2 tsp coconut oil
- 4 garlic cloves, peeled and finely sliced
- 200g green beans, trimmed and cut into 1cm pieces
- 4 tsp capers, roughly chopped
- 50g (½ cup) sun-dried tomatoes in oil, drained and sliced
- 6 tbsp pine nuts
- 2 tbsp apple cider vinegar
- 2 tbsp nutritional yeast
- 2 tsp dried basil
- pink Himalayan salt or sea salt and freshly ground black pepper
- 8 fresh basil leaves, to serve

1. Preheat the oven to 180°C/350°F/gas 4.
2. Tip the rice into a saucepan, cover with water, bring to the boil over a medium-high heat, then turn the heat down to medium-low and cook for 25 minutes or according to the packet instructions until cooked through.
3. When the rice is almost cooked, slice the peppers straight down the middle lengthways, keeping the stalks intact. Remove the seeds, place in a large baking tray, drizzle with the olive oil and roast in the hot oven for 10–15 minutes.
4. Meanwhile, heat the coconut oil in a large frying pan over a medium heat. Add the garlic, green beans, capers and sun-dried tomatoes and cook for 3-4 minutes, stirring regularly.
5. Remove from the heat, add the remaining ingredients, reserving a few pine nuts, then drain and add the cooked rice, stirring to combine.
6. Remove the peppers from the oven, stuff with the rice filling, sprinkle with the reserved pine nuts, place back in the oven and roast for 20–25 minutes. Serve with fresh basil leaves on top.

BULGUR WHEAT STUFFED COURGETTES

Serves 4

I first created this recipe when I had friends round for dinner. I had been out all day and got back late so didn't have time to make anything fancy – I put this together in 30 minutes and they loved it! Bulgur has a wonderful texture and absorbs the delicious flavours of the vegetables.

Ingredients

4 large courgettes
1 tbsp coconut oil, plus extra for the courgettes
1 corn on the cob
160g (1 cup) bulgur wheat, rinsed
1 organic low-salt vegetable stock cube
1 onion, diced
1 red pepper, deseeded and diced
5 chestnut mushrooms, finely sliced
2 garlic cloves, peeled and finely chopped
½ fresh red chilli, deseeded and finely chopped
1 tsp Cajun spice
1 tsp smoked paprika
1 tbsp apple cider vinegar
1 x Tomato Sauce recipe (see page 109)
pink Himalayan salt or sea salt and freshly ground black pepper

1. Preheat the oven to 180°C/350°F/gas 4.
2. Halve the courgettes lengthways and scoop out the seeds. Rub with a little coconut oil, place on a baking tray and bake in the hot oven for 15-20 minutes, turning halfway.
3. Boil the corn on the cob in a saucepan of boiling water for 3-5 minutes, then remove from the pan and set aside, reserving 500ml (2 cups) water. Once cooled, slice off the corn kernels.
4. Cook the bulgur wheat in the reserved water, crumbling in the stock cube. Stir and cook over a medium heat for 15 minutes, then drain and set aside.
5. Heat 1 tablespoon coconut oil in a frying pan over a medium heat and fry the onion for 5 minutes. Add all the remaining vegetables, garlic and chilli with the spices, season well with salt and black pepper, and fry for about 8 minutes.
6. Stir in the cooked bulgur wheat with the apple cider vinegar and spoon the mixture into each of the courgettes.
7. Bake for a further 5 minutes, then serve with the tomato sauce and the remaining bulgur wheat on the side.

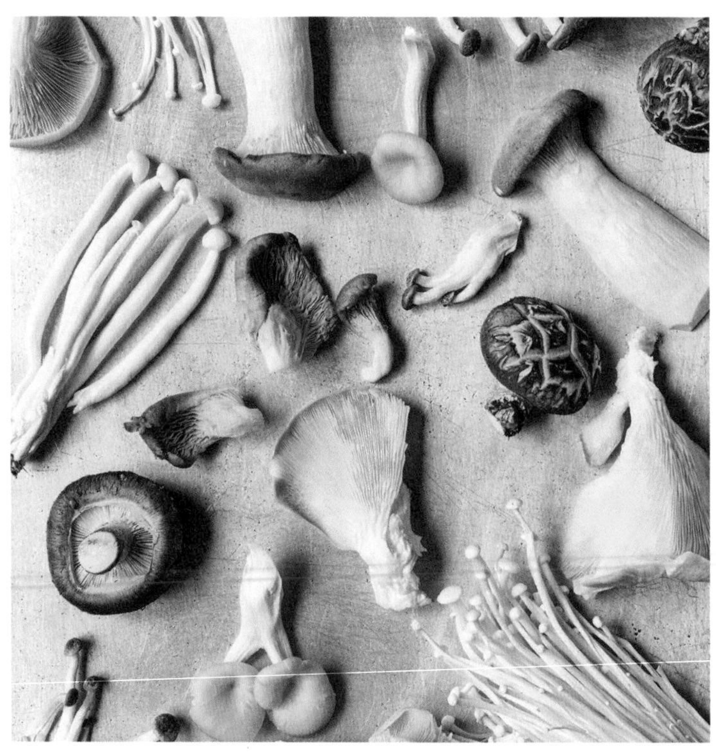

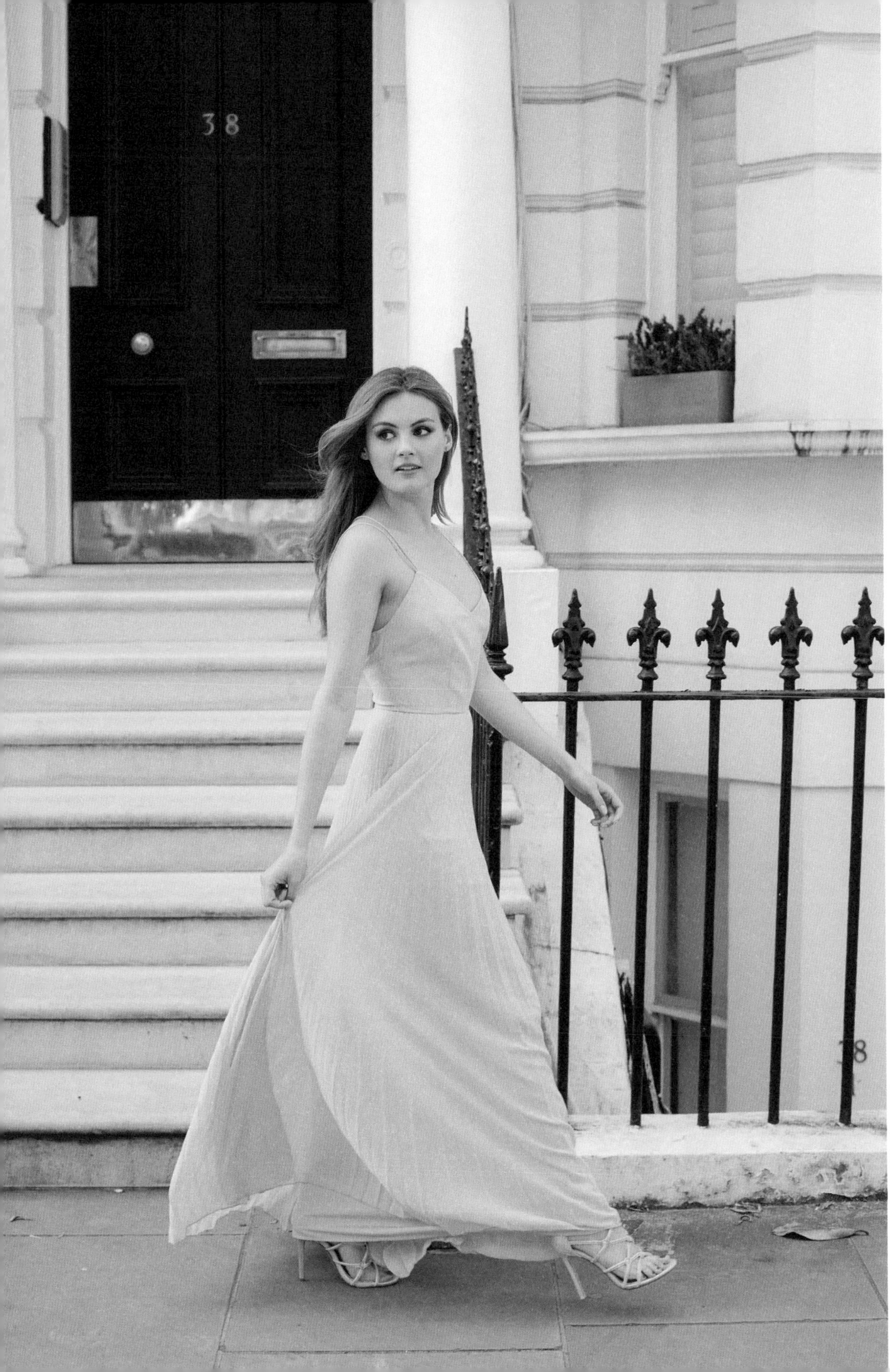

'CHEESY' PASTA BAKE

Serves 4

When I was a teenager, my speciality was pasta bake. Back then I added tinned tuna, cheese and butter, but now being on a plant-based diet I have adapted my original comfort food to make it nourishing with more sophisticated flavours. This is great to serve friends with a slice of garlic bread.

Ingredients

1 courgette, chopped
1 red pepper, deseeded and sliced
1 orange pepper, deseeded and sliced
1 onion, sliced
1 tbsp olive oil
250g (3¼ cups) brown rice pasta
1 large vine tomato, sliced
pink Himalayan salt or sea salt and freshly ground black pepper
2 tbsp pine nuts, to serve
a small handful of fresh basil leaves, chopped, to serve

spicy tomato sauce

1 garlic clove, peeled and crushed
1 tbsp olive oil
2 x 400g tins chopped tomatoes
2 tbsp tomato purée
1 tbsp mixed herbs
½ tsp dried chilli flakes
2 tbsp capers

1. Preheat the oven to 200°C/400°F/gas 6.
2. Place the vegetables in a roasting tray with a drizzle of olive oil and roast for 25 minutes.
3. Cook the pasta with a pinch of salt according to the packet instructions, then drain and set aside.
4. While the vegetables are roasting and the pasta is cooking, make the tomato sauce; fry the garlic with the olive oil in a large saucepan over a medium-high heat for a few seconds until fragrant. Add the remaining ingredients, turn the heat down to low and simmer for 15 minutes.
5. To make the 'cheese' sauce, heat the coconut oil in a small saucepan over a medium heat. Add the diced shallot and fry for 5-7 minutes to soften before adding the garlic and frying for another minute. Add 1 tablespoon of the flour and use a whisk to stir it in. Add the remaining flour, still whisking the mixture, then slowly whisk in the almond milk bit by bit.
6. Once the flour has dissolved into the almond milk, add the remaining ingredients. Continue to use the whisk to make sure there are no lumps, and then keep it on a very low heat, stirring frequently.
7. When the roasted vegetables are cooked, remove from the oven and turn the heat down to 180°C/350°F/gas 4.

'cheese' sauce
2 tsp coconut oil
1 shallot, peeled and diced
2 garlic cloves, peeled and crushed
2 tbsp buckwheat flour
250ml (1 cup) unsweetened almond milk
2 tbsp nutritional yeast
1 tbsp apple cider vinegar

garlic bread
8 garlic cloves, peeled and crushed
4 thick slices of rye or sourdough bread
4 tsp dried mixed herbs
extra-virgin olive oil
a handful of fresh basil leaves, chopped

8. Stir the roasted vegetables into the tomato sauce with the cooked pasta. Pour into a 20cm x 30cm ovenproof baking dish, pour over the 'cheese' sauce and smooth down with a spoon. Add the sliced tomato to the top and bake for 30 minutes.

9. Lightly toast the pine nuts in a dry frying pan over a medium heat and set aside.

10. To make the garlic bread, preheat the grill to medium, rub the crushed garlic onto one side of each slice of bread, sprinkle with the dried herbs and drizzle with olive oil. Grill for 5 minutes or until golden, then sprinkle with the basil.

11. Serve the pasta bake sprinkled with the toasted pine nuts and chopped basil.

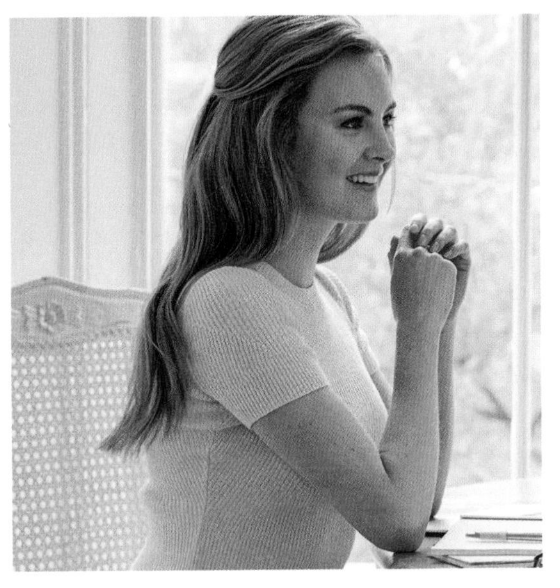

MACARONI 'CHEESE' WITH ROASTED TOMATOES

Serves 2

My family have a recipe for a creamy, cheesy pasta with tomatoes stirred through. Obviously that's not the healthiest, so I set myself the challenge to see if I could make a creamy but plant-based pasta dish. This exceeded my expectations and is now one of my favourite curl-up-on-the-sofa dinners. Get ahead by soaking your cashews overnight.

Ingredients

6 ripe vine cherry tomatoes, halved
1 tsp olive oil
a pinch of dried thyme
200g (2 cups) brown rice macaroni pasta
pink Himalayan salt or sea salt and freshly ground black pepper

'cheese' sauce

¼ small butternut squash (approx. 250g), peeled and chopped
½ small onion, diced
½ tsp coconut oil
1 garlic clove, peeled and diced
40g (¼ cup) unsalted raw cashew nuts, soaked overnight
125ml (½ cup) brown rice milk or other non-dairy milk
2 tbsp nutritional yeast
½ tsp wholegrain mustard
a pinch of ground nutmeg
juice of ½ lemon

1. Preheat the oven to 190°C/375°F/gas 5.
2. For the 'cheese' sauce, place a saucepan of boiling water over a high heat. Set a lidded steamer basket on top and steam the squash for 15 minutes until soft.
3. Meanwhile, place the tomato halves on a baking tray lined with tin foil. Drizzle with the olive oil, a sprinkling of dried thyme and a pinch of salt and pepper and roast in the hot oven for 10–15 minutes.
4. Cook the pasta according to the instructions, drain and rinse with cold water, tip back into the pan and set aside.
5. Place a frying pan over a medium heat and fry the onion for the 'cheese' sauce in the coconut oil for 5 minutes, then add the garlic and continue to fry for another minute.
6. Drain the soaked cashews and add to a high-speed blender with the steamed butternut squash, cooked onion and garlic and the remaining ingredients for the creamy sauce. Blend until totally smooth.
7. Stir into the cooked pasta and heat on a low heat for about 5 minutes to warm. Serve in bowls with the roasted tomatoes on top.

NUT WELLINGTON

Serves 4

For Christmas I wanted to make a plant-based alternative to beef Wellington and the result was outstanding! What is essentially a nut roast made from lentils, vegetables and nuts is then wrapped in thin aubergine slices. This is great for Sunday dinner, too, with roasted vegetables, mint sauce and vegetable gravy.

Ingredients

mint sauce

3 bunches of fresh mint leaves
60ml (¼ cup) apple cider vinegar
pink Himalayan salt or sea salt and freshly ground black pepper

nut Wellington

125g (½ cup) red split lentils
1 onion, diced
1 tsp coconut oil, plus extra for the aubergines
5 chestnut mushrooms, chopped
1 carrot, peeled and chopped
1 red pepper, deseeded and chopped
2 garlic cloves, peeled and diced
1 tsp dried thyme
1 tsp dried rosemary
5 sage leaves, chopped
1 tsp apple cider vinegar

1. To make the mint sauce, sprinkle a good pinch of salt onto the mint leaves, finely chop and add to a bowl or jar.
2. Stir in the apple cider vinegar and a pinch of freshly ground pepper, pour over 60ml (¼ cup) boiling water and stir.
3. Allow to cool, then refrigerate for at least 1 hour, but preferably overnight, for the flavours to infuse. Keep in an airtight jar or container in the fridge.
4. Preheat the oven to 190°C/375°F/gas 5.
5. Cook the lentils by adding to a saucepan with 1 cup of water. Bring to the boil and simmer for 15-20 minutes or until cooked.
6. Set a frying pan over a medium-high heat and fry the onion in the coconut oil for 5-7 minutes. Add the remaining vegetables and garlic, apart from the aubergine, and continue to fry for 10-15 minutes until the vegetables have softened.
7. Stir in the herbs, apple cider vinegar and season well with a pinch of salt and pepper.
8. In a food processor, pulse the mixed nuts to small chunks. Add the cooked lentils and the vegetables and blend until everything is combined, but retaining small chunks. Set aside.

(recipe continues overleaf)

125g (1 cup) mixed nuts, such as Brazil, cashew, walnuts, chopped
2 large aubergines
pink Himalayan salt or sea salt and freshly ground black pepper

9. Cut the stalks off the aubergines and cut into wide, flat 2-3mm thick slices. Some slices won't come out right, but that's why the recipe calls for 2 aubergines, to allow room for error.

10. Place on a large baking sheet, rub with coconut oil and cook in the hot oven for 10-15 minutes, turning halfway.

11. Lightly grease a 1lb loaf tin with coconut oil and place the aubergine slices around the sides of the tin, keeping them high enough for the opposite aubergine slices to be able to overlap at the top. Lay the aubergine slices along the base so the whole of the inside of the loaf tin is covered.

12. Pour in the Wellington mixture, using a wooden spoon to pack it in and smooth the top, then lay a single layer of aubergine slices on top. Fold in all the aubergine slices around the top and use toothpicks to secure the slices in place.

13. Bake on the middle shelf of the oven for 40 minutes. Remove and allow to cool slightly before removing from the tin. Pull out the toothpicks and place a chopping board on top of the tin, then flip over and gently lift the tin off.

14. Slice into four equal portions and serve with the mint sauce.

Serving ideas ...
Roasted Carrots with Thyme (see page 153).
Roasted Brussels Sprouts with Garlic (see page 153).
Rosemary-roasted Sweet Potatoes (see page 150).

Tip ... Cut any leftover aubergine into chunks and use in my Quick Quinoa (see page 142).

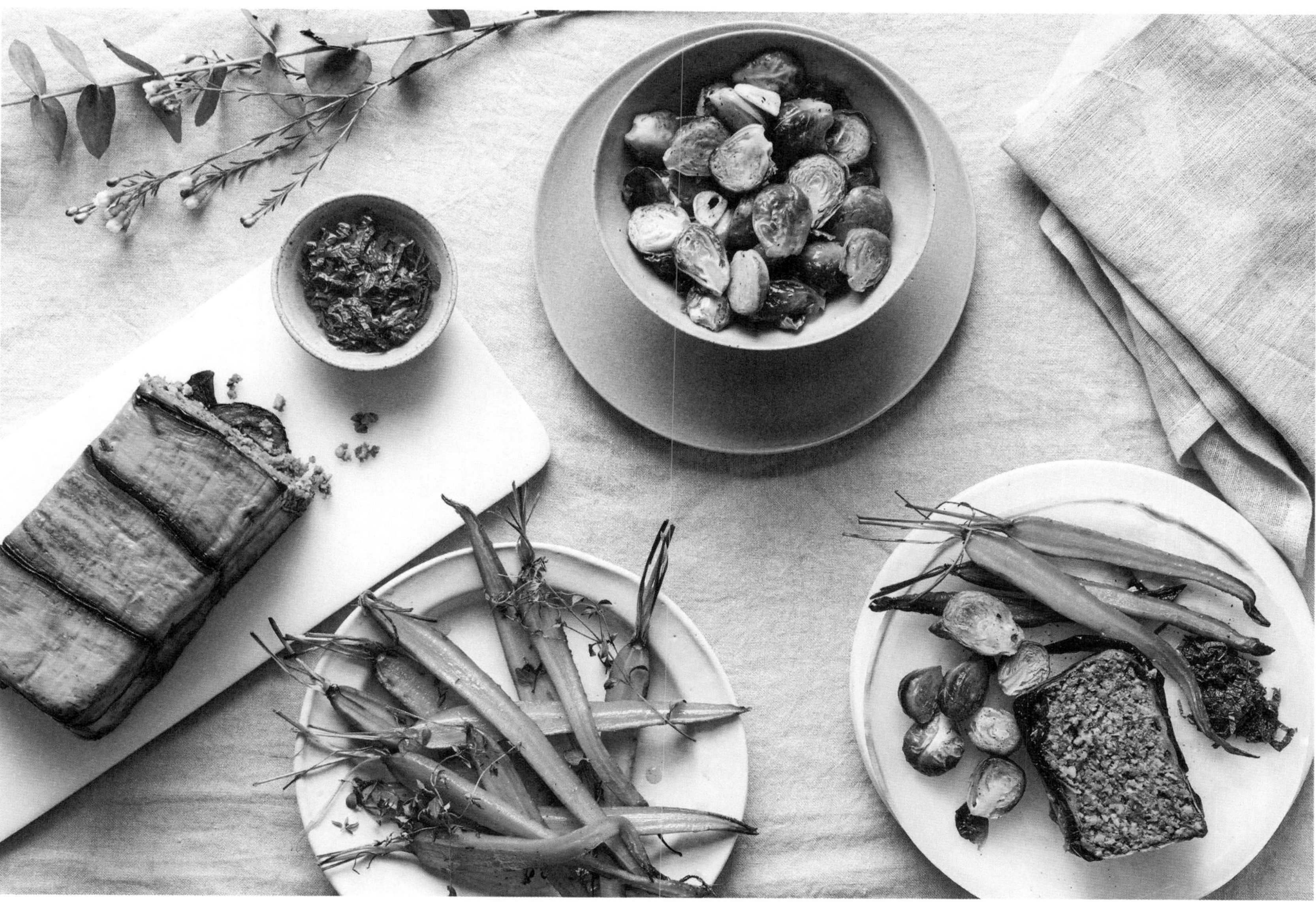

CREAMY LEEK + CELERIAC PIE

Serves 4

A hearty pie with a crisp crust and a smooth, creamy filling – who would've thought this could be possible eating plant-based? Well, I've made it possible with this absolute showstopper of a main meal. Bring this to a table of hungry family members and they will not be disappointed. Get ahead by soaking your cashews overnight.

Ingredients

1 small celeriac, peeled and chopped
olive oil
4 leeks, trimmed and sliced
1 whole broccoli, broken into small florets

sauce
150g (1 cup) unsalted raw cashew nuts, soaked overnight
300ml (2¼ cups) oat milk
1 tsp wholegrain mustard
1 tbsp nutritional yeast
1 garlic clove, peeled
a handful of fresh chives, chopped
pink Himalayan salt or sea salt and freshly ground black pepper

pastry
1 tbsp milled flaxseed
150g (1 cup) wholewheat flour
150g (1 cup) spelt flour
¼ tsp salt
60ml (¼ cup) olive oil

1. Preheat the oven to 180°C/350°F/gas 4.
2. Place the celeriac in a roasting tray, drizzle with olive oil and roast in the hot oven for 30 minutes.
3. After the 30 minutes is up, add the leeks to the celeriac and roast for a further 15 minutes.
4. Make the sauce by draining the cashews and blending in a food processor until broken apart and then add the remaining ingredients, apart from the chives, with a pinch of salt and black pepper and blend on full power for about 3 minutes until totally smooth.
5. Stir in the chopped chives and set aside while you make the pastry.
6. Mix together the flaxseed with 2 tablespoons water and set aside.
7. In a large bowl, combine both the flours and the salt. Then add the olive oil and 90ml (⅓ cup) cold water, plus more if needed, and mix together. Once thickened, add the flaxseed mixture to the bowl and use your hands to fully combine the mixture, until it all comes together.
8. Roll the dough out on a lightly floured surface to 5mm thick and 6-7cm wider than the diameter of your pie dish.

9. Combine the roasted vegetables with the broccoli and the sauce to make the filling. Spoon into the pie dish.
10. Carefully drape the pastry over the pie dish. Use your thumb and forefinger to crimp the pastry edges around the rim to seal and, using a sharp knife, make a small cross in the centre of the pastry lid.
11. Bake in the hot oven for 40–45 minutes until cooked through.

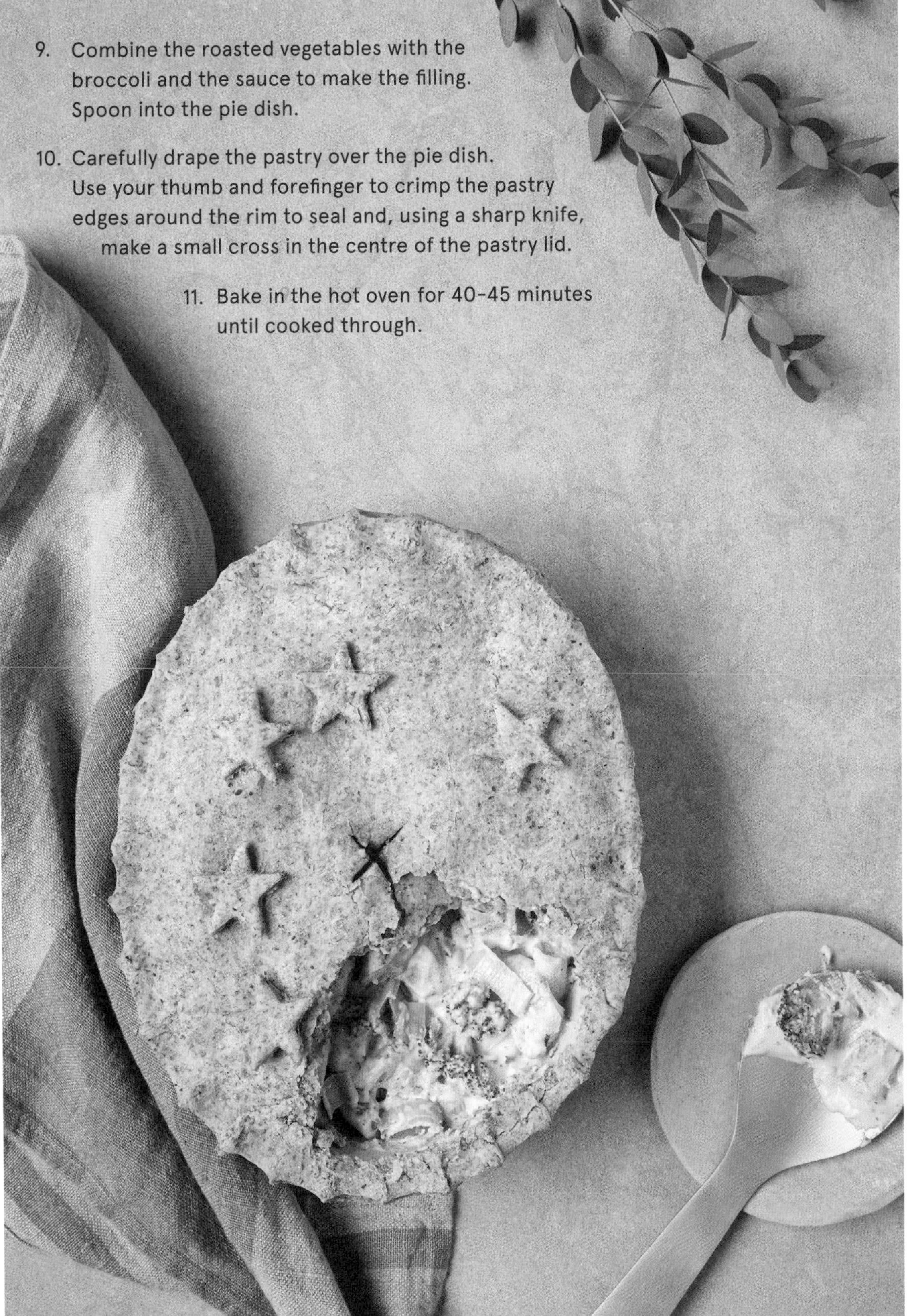

QUICK QUINOA

Serves 2

I created this recipe when I had my close friend Tanya round for dinner one evening, and I needed to make something tasty in about 30 minutes. Luckily quinoa is really quick, so I cooked it with a variety of fresh vegetables, spices and sweet dates and pomegranate. It went down a treat!

Ingredients

200g (1 cup) quinoa, rinsed
1 tbsp coconut oil
1 red onion, diced
½ tsp turmeric
½ tsp ground cinnamon
1 tsp ground cumin
1 aubergine, cubed
10 ripe vine cherry tomatoes, quartered
1 yellow pepper, deseeded and diced
1 x 400g tin chopped tomatoes
½ fresh red chilli, deseeded and diced
2 medjool dates, pitted and diced
a large handful of spinach
½ pomegranate, seeded
a bunch of fresh coriander, leaves picked and chopped
pink Himalayan salt or sea salt and freshly ground black pepper

1. Tip the quinoa into a saucepan with 500ml (2 cups) of water. Place over a medium heat, bring to the boil, then turn the heat down to low and simmer for 15 minutes until the water has been absorbed and the quinoa is cooked, adding more water if needed. Keep to one side.
2. Heat half of the coconut oil in a frying pan over a medium heat, add the onion and fry for 5 minutes until softened.
3. Add the spices, fry for a further couple of minutes, then add the aubergine and fry this for about 10 minutes, until softened, adding more coconut oil if needed.
4. Add the cherry tomatoes and pepper with a pinch of salt and black pepper and fry for a further 5 minutes.
5. Add the tinned tomatoes, chilli and dates, bring to a simmer.
6. Remove from the heat, stir in the spinach and quinoa and serve sprinkled with the pomegranate seeds and the chopped coriander.

Tip ... Save any leftover pomegranate seeds and sprinkle over a bowl of homemade Muesli (see page 48), for breakfast.

ITALIAN FARRO + BEAN STEW

Serves 4

Whenever I think of stews, I'm reminded of my great grandmother, who made them for all the family, usually with beef and dumplings. I used to love it as a kid, so I wanted to create a healthier version that I can enjoy – and this is the delicious result.

Ingredients

olive oil
1 onion, diced
2 carrots, peeled and diced
1 organic low-salt vegetable stock cube
50g (½ cup) farro, rinsed
½ fresh red chilli, peeled and chopped
1 garlic clove, peeled and diced
1 x 400g tin chopped tomatoes
1 x 400g tin cannellini beans, drained
1 lemon
2 tbsp nutritional yeast (optional)
150g (3 packed cups) spinach
½ bunch of fresh basil leaves, chopped
pink Himalayan salt or sea salt and freshly ground black pepper

1. Heat a little olive oil in a large saucepan over a medium heat. Add the onion and fry for 5 minutes until softened, stirring occasionally, then add the carrot and fry for another 3 minutes.

2. Dissolve the stock cube in 750ml (3 cups) boiling water in a jug and keep to one side.

3. Add the farro, chilli and garlic to the carrots and fry for a further minute, stirring regularly, before adding the stock and chopped tomatoes.

4. Bring to the boil, then turn the heat down to medium-low and simmer for 30 minutes, stirring occasionally.

5. After 30 minutes, stir in the beans, squeeze in the lemon juice, add the nutritional yeast, if using, and simmer for a further 5 minutes to warm through.

6. Season to taste with salt and pepper and, just before serving, stir in the spinach until wilted. Serve sprinkled with the basil.

Tip ... Make this recipe and freeze any leftover portions to defrost and eat another day.

SPRING GARDEN RISOTTO

Serves 4

When I first started cooking, I used to avoid making risotto because I thought it was too complicated, with the constant stirring and watching over it, but when I tried it out one day I realised how easy it can be. I love the taste of spring from the wonderful greens in this.

Ingredients

1 organic low-salt vegetable stock cube
2 shallots, peeled and diced
1 tbsp olive oil
juice of 1 lemon
300g (1½ cups) brown risotto rice or arborio rice
1 carrot, peeled and diced
½ courgette, diced
175g (¼ cup) fresh, frozen or tinned broad beans
80g (½ cup) frozen peas
a small bunch of asparagus, woody ends removed and thinly sliced
2 spring onions, trimmed and finely sliced
1 tbsp nutritional yeast
¼ bunch of fresh mint, leaves picked and chopped
pink Himalayan salt or sea salt and freshly ground black pepper
a handful of watercress, to serve

1. Dissolve the stock cube in 1.5 litres (6 cups) boiling water in a saucepan over a low heat.
2. Place a frying pan over a medium-low heat and fry the shallots in the olive oil for 5 minutes until softened. Add half the lemon juice with the rice and fry for another 2 minutes.
3. Add the carrot with the remaining lemon juice and fry for a further 3-5 minutes.
4. Add one ladle of the veg stock to the pan and keep stirring until the rice has absorbed all the liquid. Repeat this for 25 minutes or according to the instructions on the packet of rice, adding one ladle of stock at a time and continuously stirring.
5. For the final 10 minutes, add the courgette, broad beans, peas, asparagus and spring onions. When the last of the stock has been absorbed, season well with salt and pepper and remove from the heat. Stir in the nutritional yeast and most of the mint.
6. Serve sprinkled with the remaining mint and with a handful of watercress on top.

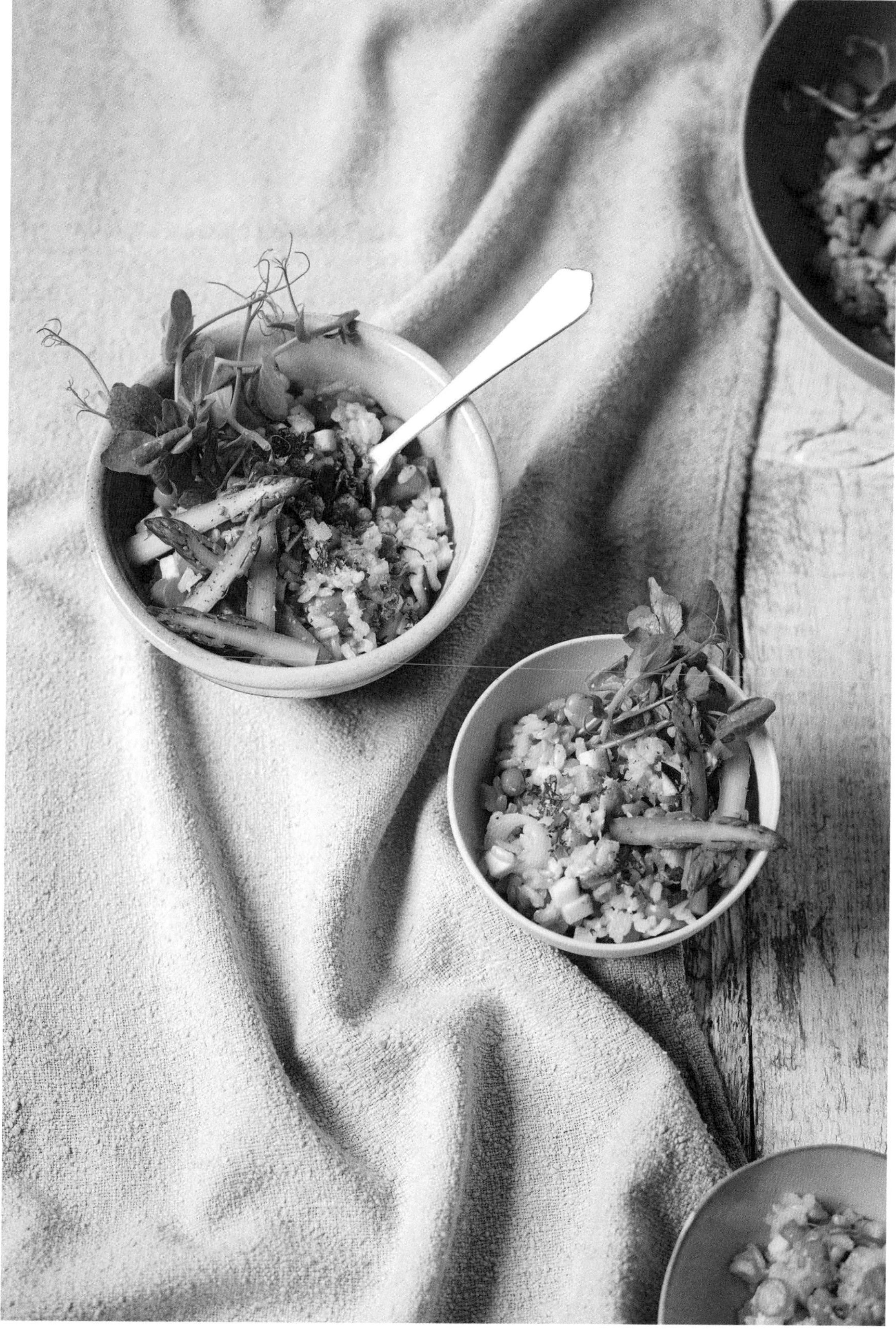

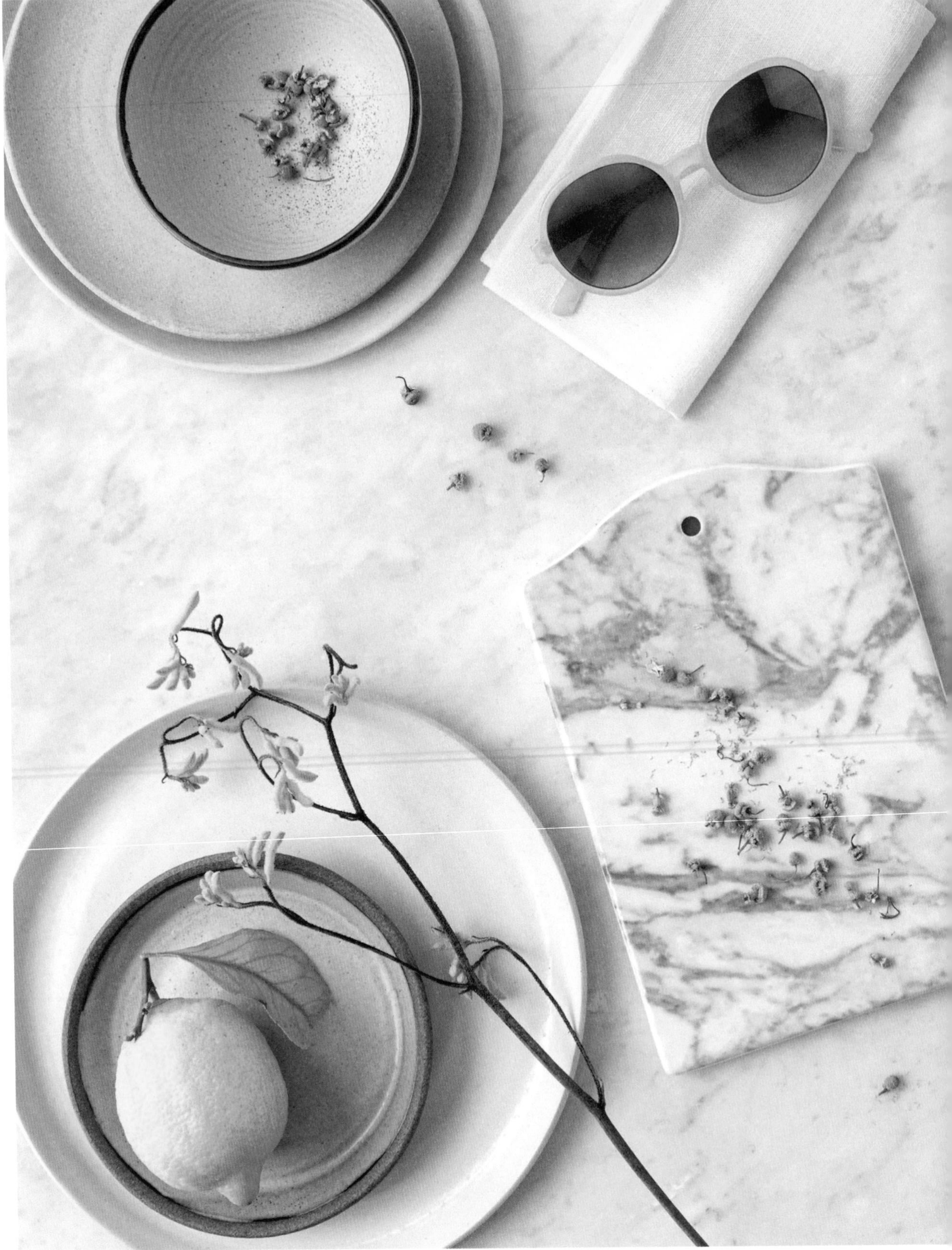

Sides + Snacks

04

ROASTED MEDITERRANEAN VEGETABLES

Serves 4

I spent a lot of my childhood in Mallorca and loved the way the abundance of local vegetables were used. So these two recipes call for simply roasting a variety of vegetables to make tasty side dishes. I first discovered roasting whole garlic at a restaurant called The Stinking Rose in LA, where everything includes garlic. My kind of restaurant! I love this spread over crackers or to serve at dinner parties.

SPANISH-STYLE

Serves 4

Ingredients

1 red pepper, deseeded
1 yellow pepper, deseeded
2 red onions
2 courgettes
2 garlic cloves, unpeeled
1 tbsp coconut oil or olive oil
125g (1 cup) cherry tomatoes
1 tsp mixed dried herbs
pink Himalayan salt or sea salt and freshly ground black pepper

1. Preheat the oven to 190°C/375°F/gas 5.
2. Slice the peppers and onions into strips and the courgettes into discs. Cut the garlic cloves in half.
3. If using coconut oil, place in a large roasting tray in the oven until melted before adding the vegetables.
4. Scatter the mixed herbs over the vegetables and make sure everything is covered evenly in the oil, then season with salt and black pepper. Roast in the hot oven for 45 minutes, checking every 15 minutes that the vegetables are not burning and are cooking evenly.

WHOLE ROASTED GARLIC

Serves 4

Ingredients

1 large whole garlic bulb
olive oil
rye bread or crackers, to serve

1. Preheat the oven to 190°C/375°F/gas 5.
2. Remove the loose outer layers of the garlic and cut off the top – enough to slice the tops off the individual cloves.
3. Place on a sheet of tin foil and drizzle with olive oil. Wrap up in the foil and roast in the hot oven for 45 minutes.
4. Serve spread onto rye bread, crackers or Rosemary Crackers (see page 166).

SWEET POTATOES

Serves 4

Sweet potato is probably my favourite vegetable, and when I first made these wedges I became a little obsessed! They are perfect dipped into Homemade Ketchup (see page 154) and are a lunchtime staple. The rosemary roasted sweet potatoes are a great alternative to the traditional roasted spuds to accompany a roast dinner.

SPICED WEDGES

Serves 4

Ingredients

2-3 sweet potatoes (approx. 800g)
olive oil
1 tbsp Cajun spice
pink Himalayan salt or sea salt and freshly ground black pepper

1. Preheat the oven to 180°C/350°F/gas 4.
2. Cut the sweet potato into wedges, trying to keep all the wedges the same size so they cook evenly.
3. Place in a large roasting tray, drizzle over some olive oil and sprinkle with the spice and seasoning. Mix up with your hands or a spatula to make sure all the wedges are covered and try to lay out all the wedges so they don't overlap.
4. Roast in the hot oven for 1 hour, turning twice throughout cooking. It's good to occasionally check on them, particularly near the end of the cooking time, to make sure they're not too overdone.

Tip ... Try swapping the Cajun spice for 1 teaspoon smoked paprika and 1 teaspoon dried mixed herbs for a twist.

ROSEMARY-ROASTED

Serves 4

Ingredients

2 large sweet potatoes, peeled and chopped into 4cm chunks
2 tbsp coconut oil
2 tbsp nutritional yeast
6 sprigs of fresh rosemary (3 whole, 3 with leaves picked)
pink Himalayan salt or sea salt and freshly ground black pepper

1. Preheat the oven to 190°C/375°F/gas 5. Cover the sweet potatoes with water in a large saucepan. Bring to the boil and simmer for 8 minutes. Then drain.
2. Add 1 tablespoon of the oil along with a pinch of salt, pepper and the nutritional yeast. Place the lid on the saucepan and gently shake the potatoes to fluff up edges. This will give them a crispier finish.
3. Add the remaining coconut oil to a roasting tray and place in the oven for a few seconds to melt.
4. Add the potatoes with the whole rosemary sprigs and season. Scatter over the rosemary leaves. Roast for 45-50 minutes, until nicely browned. Remove the whole rosemary sprigs before serving.

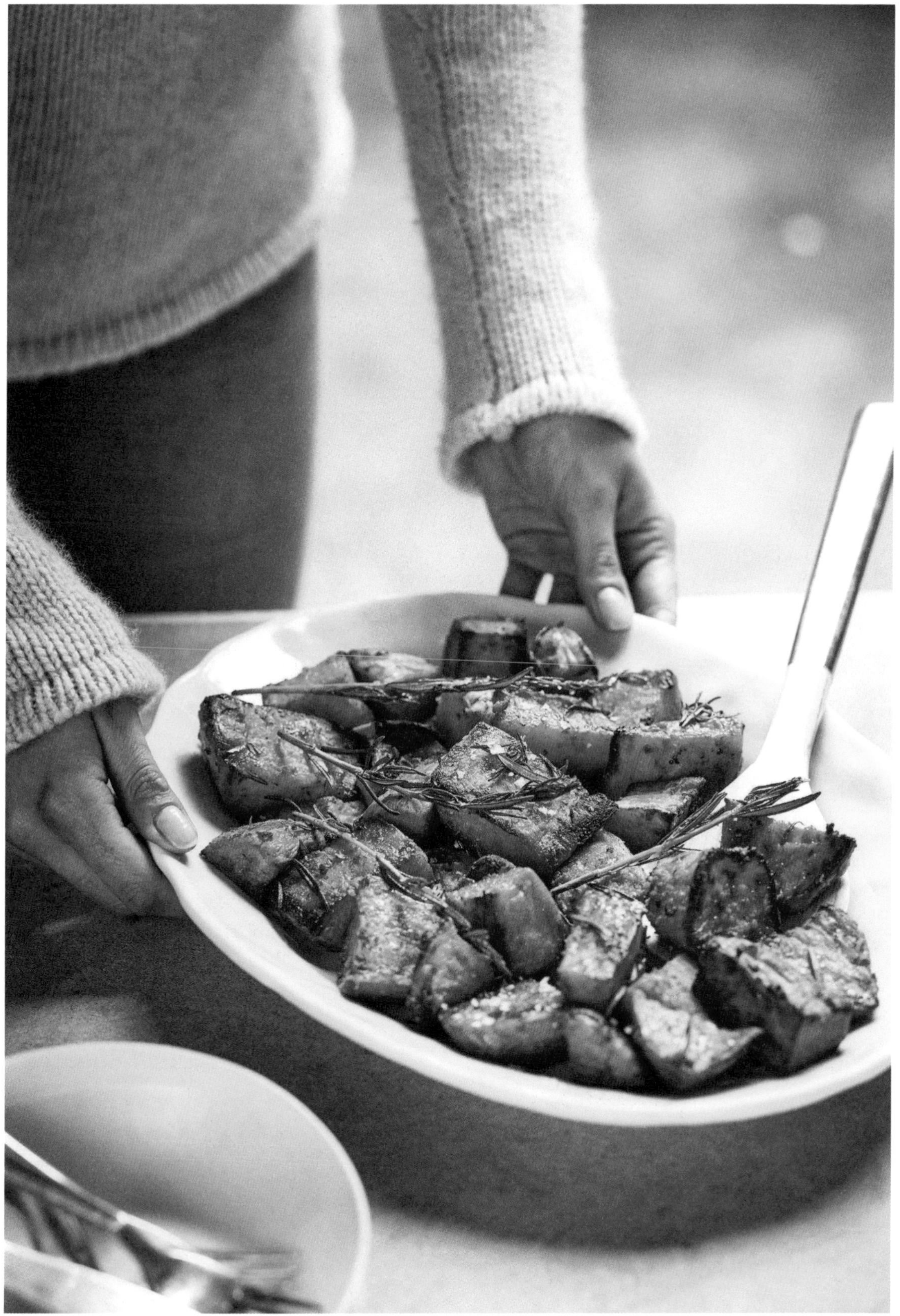

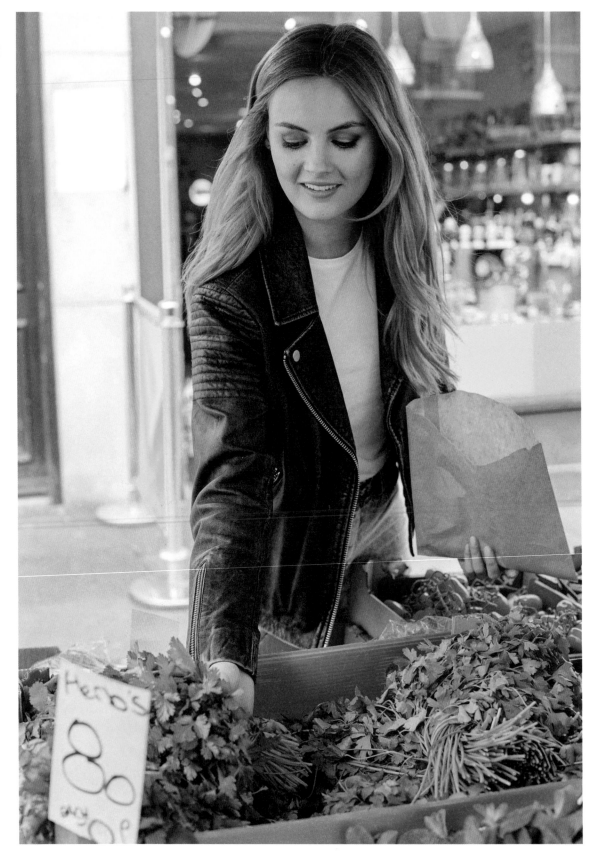
Herb's
80

SUNDAY-LUNCH SIDES

Sunday lunch can be a rather monumental time for food, often involving vegetables roasted in lashings of butter, goose fat or oil. My version uses coconut oil to roast the veggies and give them a wonderful crisp surface and mild taste. I serve these with my Nut Wellington (see page 137).

ROASTED CARROTS WITH THYME

Serves 4

Ingredients

1 tbsp coconut oil
6 fresh thyme sprigs
12 long, thin carrots, peeled and halved lengthways, leafy tops intact
pink Himalayan salt or sea salt and freshly ground black pepper

1. Preheat the oven to 190°C /375°F/gas 5.
2. While the oven is warming, put the coconut oil into a roasting tray and place in the oven to melt.
3. Pick and roughly chop half the thyme leaves. Place the carrots in the roasting tray with the 3 whole thyme sprigs, the chopped thyme and a pinch of salt and black pepper.
4. Toss everything together in the coconut oil, making sure all the carrots are evenly covered, and roast in the hot oven for 35-40 minutes, until cooked through and golden, turning over halfway.

ROASTED BRUSSELS SPROUTS WITH GARLIC

Serves 4

Ingredients

1 tbsp coconut oil
3 large handfuls of Brussels sprouts (about 20)
4 garlic cloves, peeled and finely sliced
pink Himalayan salt or sea salt and freshly ground black pepper

1. Preheat the oven to 190°C /375°F/gas 5.
2. While the oven is warming, add the coconut oil to a roasting tray and place in the oven. Remove when it has melted and set aside.
3. Rinse and dry the Brussels sprouts, slice off the stems and cut in half. Add to the roasting tray with salt and pepper, making sure the Brussels sprouts are fully covered, and roast for 10 minutes.
4. Add the garlic cloves to the roasting tray and roast for a further 10 minutes.

HOMEMADE TOMATO KETCHUP

Ketchup is one of two things that most people automatically buy at supermarkets and don't consider making at home, but it tastes so much fresher and of course doesn't contain lots of added sugar. It's easy to make and any leftovers can be used as a pasta sauce.

Ingredients

2 shallots, peeled and finely diced
1 garlic clove, peeled and crushed
1 tsp coconut oil
5 large ripe vine tomatoes, roughly chopped
1 tsp runny honey (or other sweetener)
1 tbsp apple cider vinegar
½ tsp ground cinnamon
½ tsp dried basil

1. To make the ketchup, fry the shallots and garlic in a medium saucepan over a medium-high heat with the coconut oil until golden, stirring regularly.
2. Add the chopped tomatoes to the saucepan, then turn the heat down to low and cook for 7-10 minutes until the tomatoes start to break down and soften. Stir to make sure they don't burn.
3. Add the remaining ingredients and use a wooden spoon to mash the tomatoes down.
4. Simmer for 15 minutes, then remove from the heat and set aside to cool.
5. Transfer to a blender and blend until smooth. Keep in the fridge in an airtight container for 2–3 days.

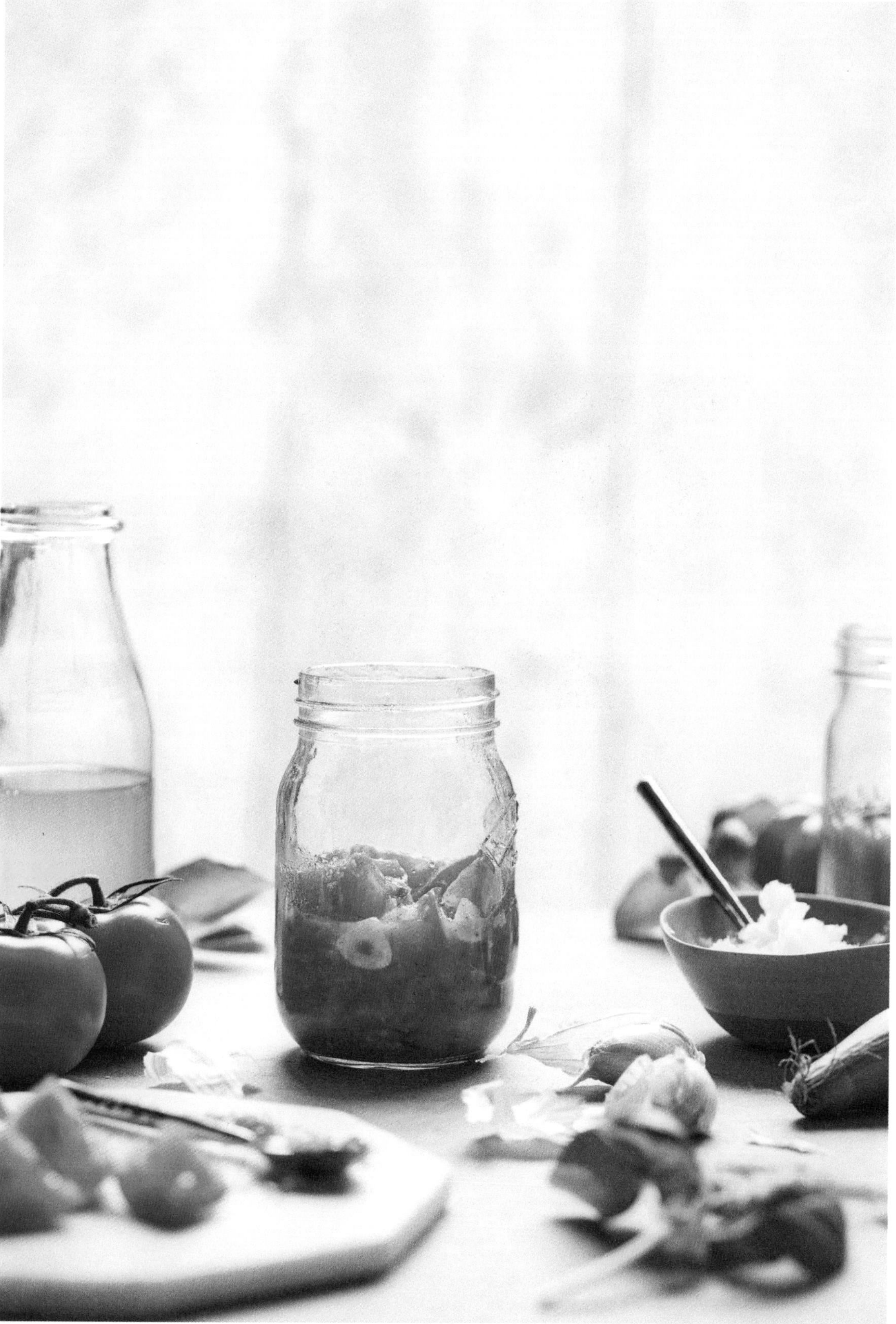

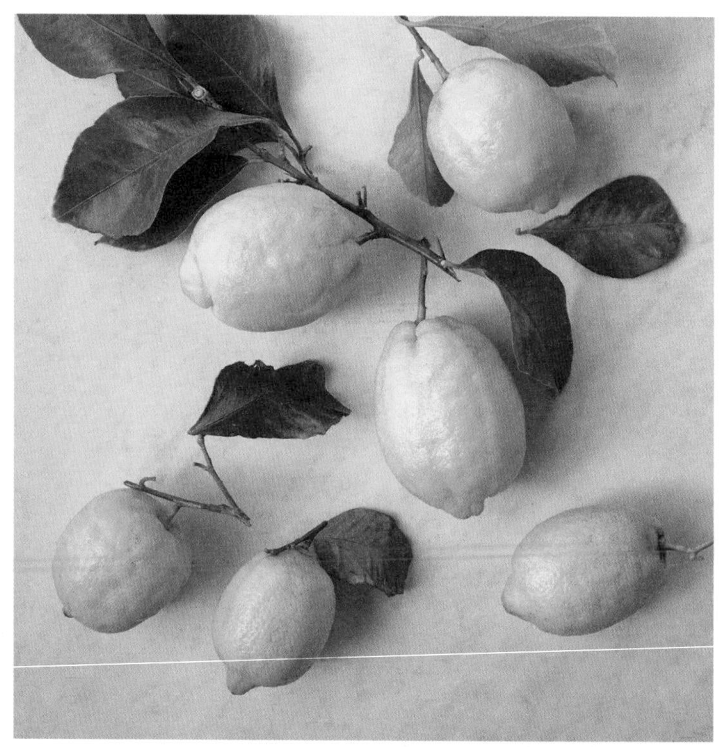

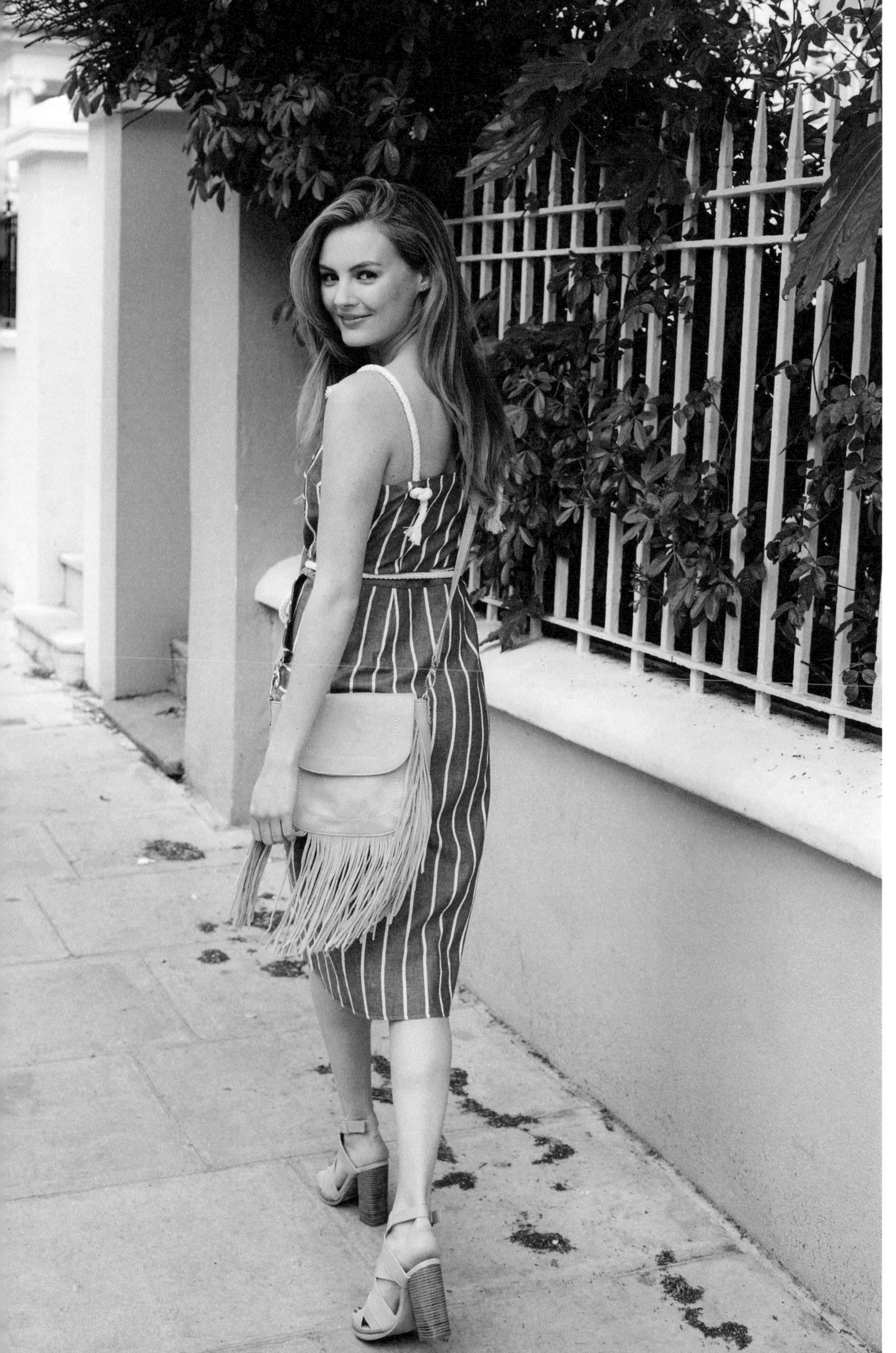

STAPLE SIDES

The dips on this page are inspired by Mexican cuisine, using chilli and fresh coriander. They're refreshing, zingy and slightly spicy, working perfectly when paired together. The salsa will keep in the fridge but the guacamole needs to be made just before eating, as the avocado will turn brown. Pesto is a real staple and so versatile and the cashew cheese I serve with almost anything. It's so delicious. Soaking the nuts overnight softens them to give a smoother consistency.

SUMMER SALSA

Ingredients

250g (2 cups) ripe vine cherry tomatoes
¼ red onion
juice of ½ lime
1 tbsp extra-virgin olive oil
½ fresh red chilli, deseeded
a handful of fresh coriander leaves
¼ cucumber, deseeded and chopped into small chunks
pink Himalayan salt or sea salt and freshly ground black pepper

1. Place the tomatoes, onion, lime juice, olive oil, chilli and seasoning into a food processor and pulse until the tomatoes and onion are chopped to the consistency that you would like the salsa. If there is a lot of liquid from the tomatoes, spoon out the excess.
2. Stir the coriander leaves into the salsa with the cucumber chunks.

Tip ... If you don't have a food processor, simply finely dice the ingredients instead.

Serving ideas ...
Mexican Chilli Bowl (see page 99).

GUACAMOLE

Ingredients

1 ripe avocado, peeled and stoned
5 ripe vine cherry tomatoes
½ fresh red chilli, deseeded
juice of ½ lime
¼ bunch of fresh coriander, leaves picked
pink Himalayan salt or sea salt and freshly ground black pepper

1. Use the back of a fork to mash the avocado and set aside.
2. Quarter the tomatoes and slice the chilli and stir into the mashed avocado with the remaining ingredients. Serve immediately.

BASIL PESTO

Ingredients

a large bunch of fresh basil, leaves picked
60g (½ cup) pumpkin seeds
80g (½ cup) pine nuts, plus 1 tbsp extra
juice of ½ lemon
2 garlic cloves, peeled
2 tbsp nutritional yeast
60ml (¼ cup) olive oil
pink Himalayan salt or sea salt and freshly ground black pepper

1. Simply place all the ingredients apart from a few basil leaves into a blender or food processor with a pinch of salt and black pepper (I use a NutriBullet with the milling blade) and process until smooth.

Tip ... Once you've made this recipe, you can experiment with different combinations of nuts and herbs here, too, such as walnuts, almonds, Brazil nuts, cashews, and you can even swap the herbs for parsley or coriander.

Serving ideas ...
Stir into squash spaghetti and top with toasted seeds and basil leaves.
Toss through a salad as a dressing.

CASHEW CHEESE

Ingredients

150g (1 cup) unsalted raw cashew nuts, soaked overnight
1 garlic clove, peeled and chopped
2 tbsp lemon juice
3 tbsp nutritional yeast
pink Himalayan salt or sea salt and freshly ground black pepper

1. Drain the cashews and place in a food processor with 125ml (¼ cup) of water and the remaining ingredients.

2. Pulse until the cashews break down, then blend for a couple of minutes until smooth and season to taste.

ROOT CRISPS

If you're tempted by the packet of crisps you know is hiding at the back of the cupboard, reach for vegetables instead. You may not think they'll satisfy the craving, but these bright, beautiful veggie crisps taste incredible when baked. They're also surprisingly quick and easy to whip up, too!

Ingredients

3-5 root vegetables, such as sweet potato, purple potato, white potato, carrot, parsnip, beetroot
1 tbsp olive oil
pink Himalayan salt or sea salt

Flavour options

1 tsp dried mixed herbs, smoked paprika, dried chilli flakes, ground cumin, dried thyme, dried rosemary

1. Preheat the oven to 160°C/310°F/gas 2½.
2. Using the slicing side of a box grater, finely slice all the vegetables. Alternatively, you can finely slice by hand or in a food processor.
3. Pat the vegetables dry on kitchen paper and add to a large bowl with the olive oil, salt and any flavourings you may like (see ingredients list for my favourites). Mix with your hands until evenly coated, then transfer onto baking sheets without overlapping.
4. Cook in the hot oven for 20-25 minutes until golden and crispy. Some may cook quicker than others, so keep an eye on them. Remove from the oven and leave to cool.

Serving ideas ...

Try with a selection of my dips (see pages 162–3).

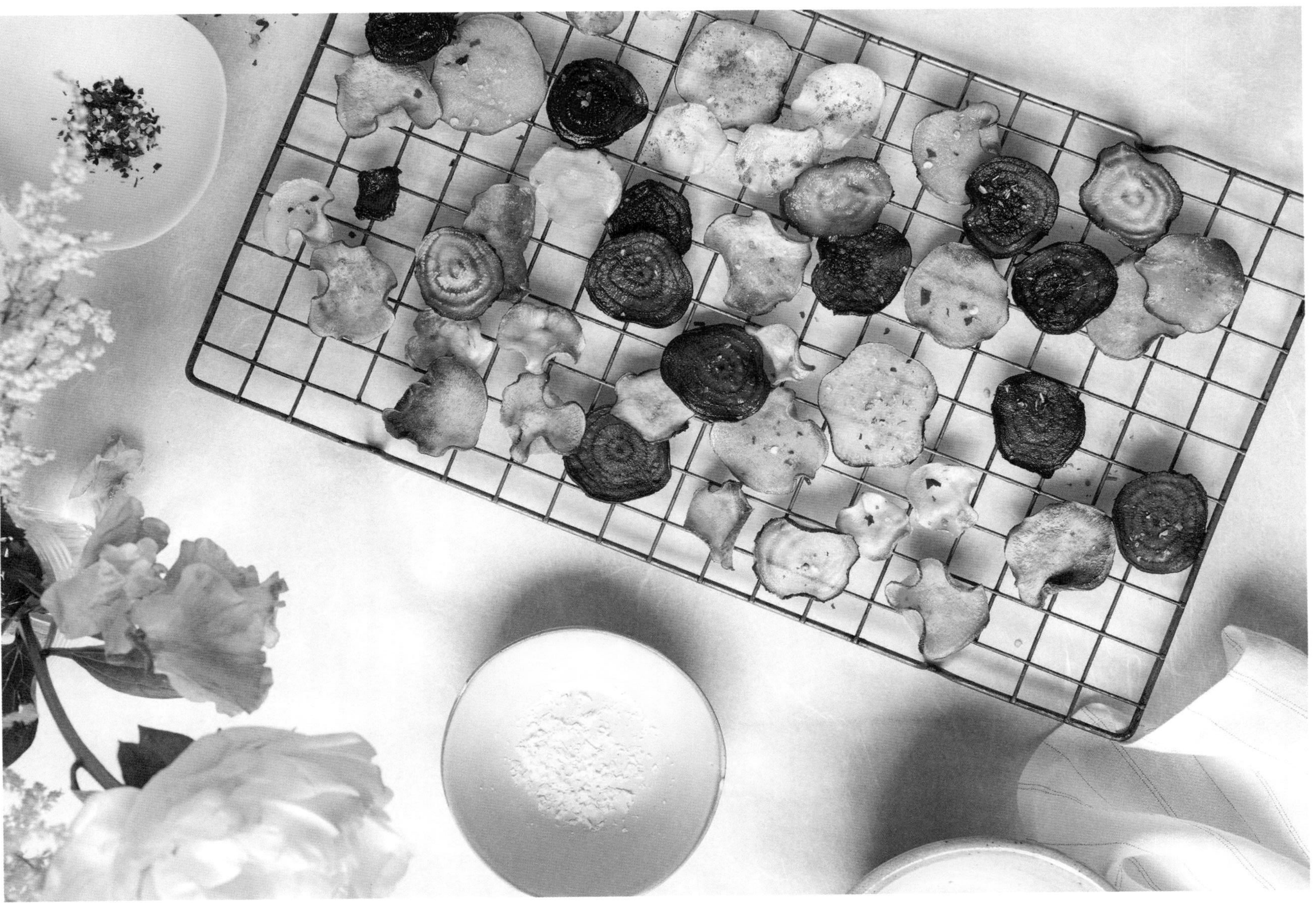

HOUMOUS – 3 WAYS

I can quite proudly say that I am a self-confessed dip addict! These dips can be enjoyed with crackers, vegetable crudités or with a salad. As I'm such a huge houmous fan I've created three delicious but very different flavours.

CLASSIC

Ingredients

1 x 400g tin chickpeas, drained
2 garlic cloves, peeled
juice of 1 lemon
3 tbsp tahini
1 tsp ground cumin
3 tbsp extra-virgin olive oil, plus extra to serve
pink Himalayan salt or sea salt and freshly ground black pepper

1. Pulse the chickpeas and garlic cloves together for 1 minute in a food processor, then add the rest of the ingredients along with a pinch of salt and pepper and a splash of water until smooth and whizz. Serve drizzled with extra-virgin olive oil.

PINK BEETROOT

Ingredients

1 x 400g tin chickpeas, drained
2 garlic cloves, peeled
1 beetroot, roughly chopped
juice of 1 lemon
2 tbsp tahini
3 tbsp extra-virgin olive oil
pink Himalayan salt or sea salt and freshly ground black pepper

1. Pulse the chickpeas and garlic cloves together for 1 minute in a food processor, then add the rest of the ingredients with a pinch of salt and pepper and a splash of water and whizz until smooth.

PEA + MINT

Ingredients

300g (2 cups) peas, fresh or frozen
2 spring onions, trimmed
10 fresh mint leaves
2 tbsp tahini
1 tbsp extra-virgin olive oil
zest and juice of ½ lemon
pink Himalayan salt or sea salt and freshly ground black pepper

1. Cook the peas in a saucepan of boiling water for about 3 minutes, then drain.
2. Finely slice half a spring onion and set aside.
3. Add the peas to a food processor with the remaining 1½ spring onions, the mint, a splash of water, the tahini, olive oil and lemon juice.
4. Whizz to your desired consistency, I like it to be quite chunky.
5. Keep in the fridge until ready to serve, then sprinkle with the lemon zest and the sliced spring onion.

DIPS

The nutritional yeast in my Sun-dried Tomato + Cashew dip gives it a cheesy flavour, but is totally optional. Spread the dip over a portobello mushroom and grill for a few minutes, stir into a pasta, or simply add to the side of any dish as a delicious dip. You can stir in the hemp seeds after blending if you like – I love doing this because they almost pop in your mouth. The Black Bean dip makes a great side to any Mexican dish – try it with my Mexican Chilli Bowl (see page 99).

BLACK BEAN

Ingredients

2 x 400g tins black beans, drained
juice of 1 lime
1 garlic clove, peeled and crushed
a small bunch of fresh coriander, leaves picked
2 tsp ground cumin
½ tsp dried chilli flakes
1 tsp smoked paprika
2–3 tbsp tinned coconut milk
pink Himalayan salt or sea salt and freshly ground black pepper

1. Add all the ingredients to a large bowl with a pinch of salt and pepper and use a hand blender (or food processor) to blend it all together. It doesn't have to be totally smooth, it can have a few pieces of beans!

2. Taste and season with a little more salt and black pepper, if needed. If you like it creamier, add more coconut milk.

Tip ... If you don't have a food processor, use a fork to mash the ingredients together.

SUN-DRIED TOMATO + CASHEW

Ingredients

150g (1 cup) unsalted raw cashew nuts
75g (½ cup) sun-dried tomatoes
2 garlic cloves, peeled
40g (¼ cup) hemp seeds
a drizzle of extra virgin olive oil
a squeeze of lime juice
1 tbsp nutritional yeast (optional)
freshly ground black pepper

1. Add all the ingredients to a food processor with 125ml (½ cup) water and blend to your desired consistency, adding more water if needed. I whizz mine up for about 3 minutes so that the cashews have broken down, but the mixture isn't too smooth.

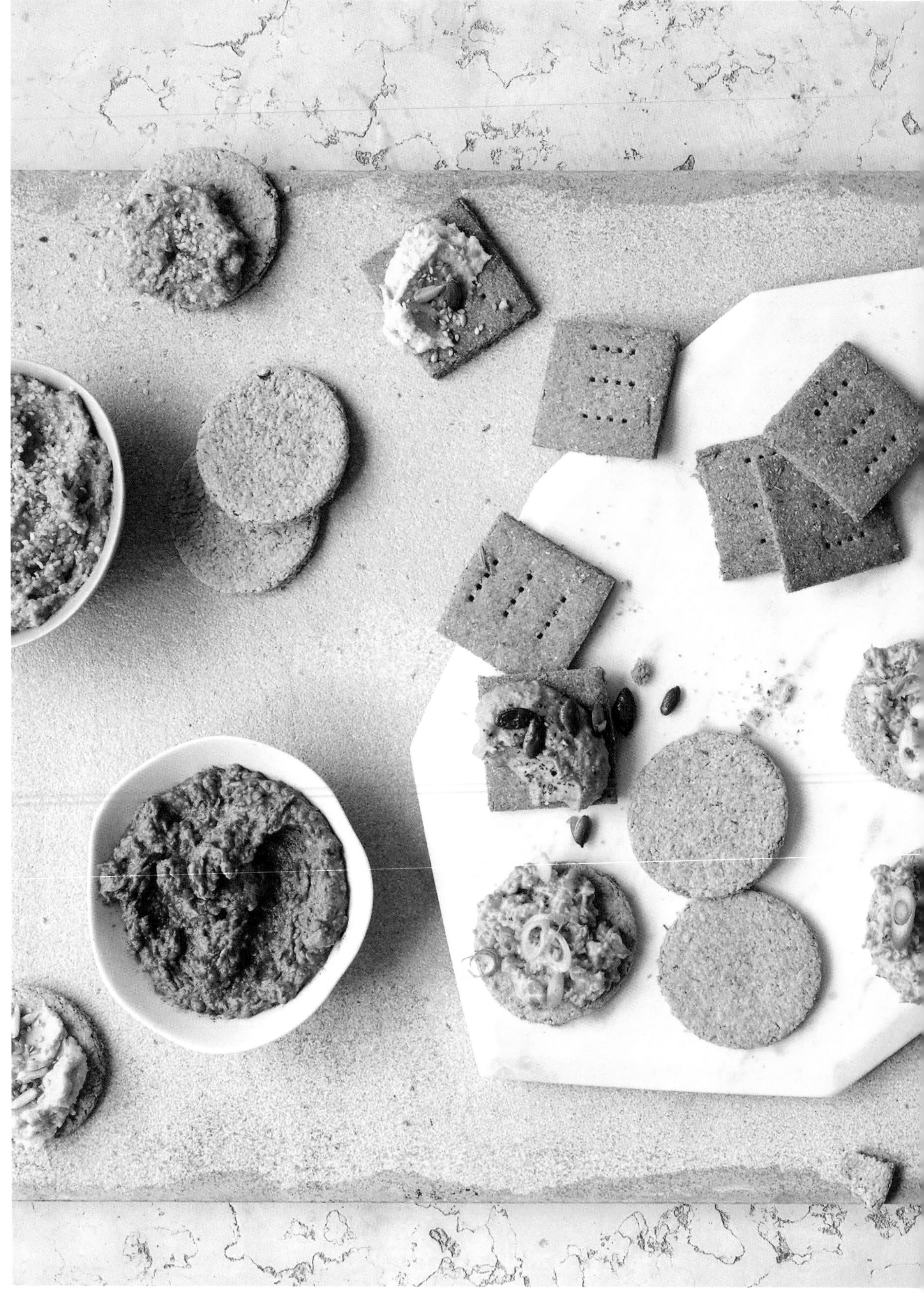

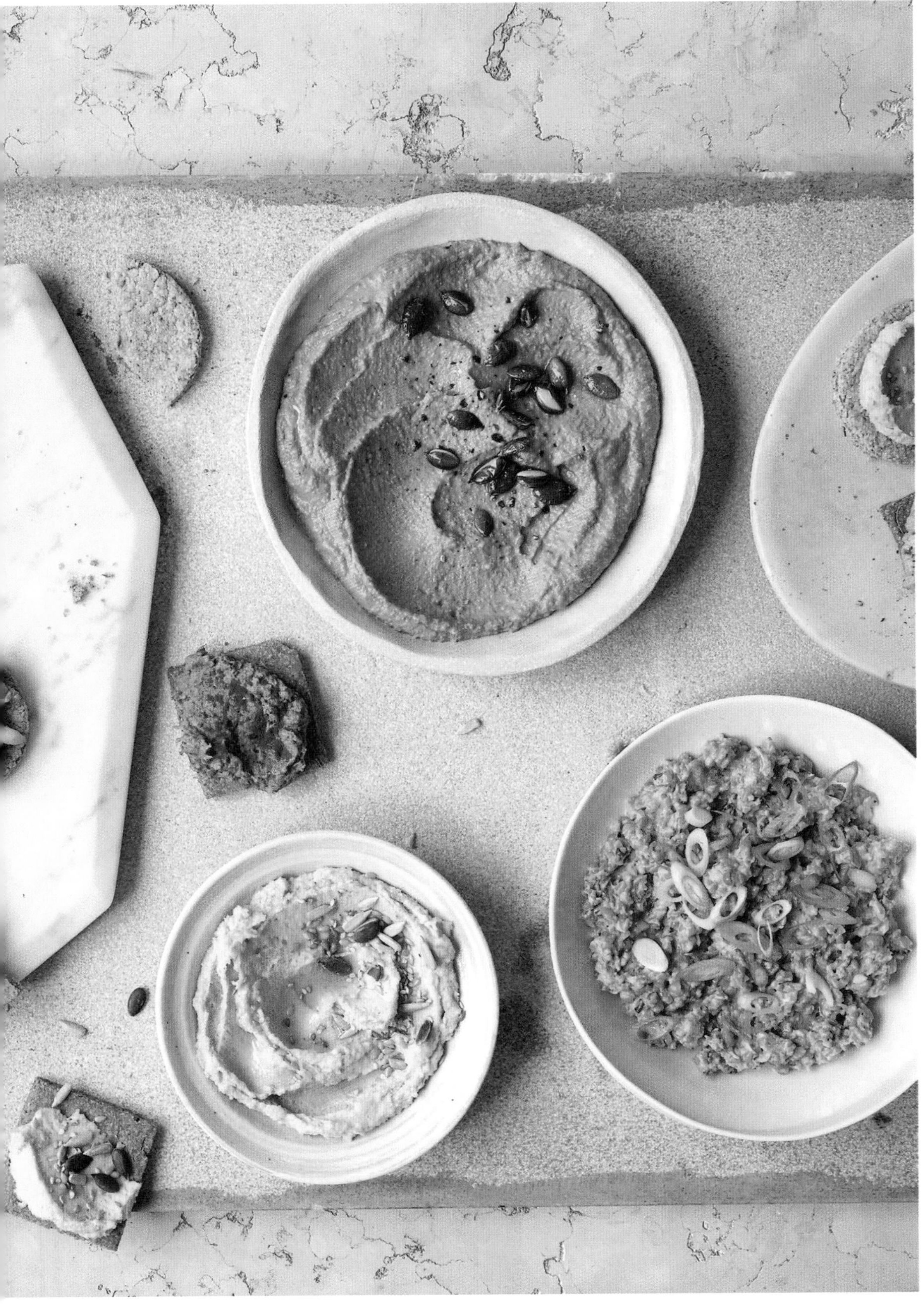

ROSEMARY CRACKERS

Makes 30

Crackers are usually relatively plain, so that whatever you pair them with will really stand out, but I love that my rosemary crackers are flavoured with onion, garlic and, of course, one of my favourite herbs, rosemary, so that they're tasty enough to enjoy on their own.

Ingredients

100g (1 cup) maize flour, plus extra for dusting
150g (1½ cups) rye flour, plus extra for dusting
½ tsp onion powder
¼ tsp garlic powder
1½ tsp dried rosemary
½ tsp pink Himalayan salt or sea salt
½ tsp freshly ground black pepper
½ tsp bicarbonate of soda
60ml (¼ cup) olive oil

1. Preheat the oven to 170°C/325°F/gas 3. Line two baking sheets with greaseproof paper.
2. Mix the flours together in a large bowl with the remaining dry ingredients.
3. Pour in the olive oil and mix until crumbly, then stir in 100ml (⅓ cup) water and mix to form a dough.
4. Roll out the dough on a floured surface until about 2.5mm-5mm thick. Slice into evenly sized squares (about 5-6cm x 5-6cm) and use a fork to prick each cracker three times.
5. Place on the lined baking sheets and bake in the hot oven for 30 minutes, until crisp and golden, turning halfway.
6. Allow to cool and keep in an airtight container.

OAT CAKES

Makes 18

If you aren't too familiar with oat cakes, they're quite simply crackers made predominantly from oats. Their mild flavour means they make a great accompaniment to a variety of sweet or savoury dips and spreads, such as houmous or almond butter.

Ingredients

225g (2¼ cups) rolled oats
½ tsp bicarbonate of soda
1 tsp dried oregano
2 tbsp extra-virgin olive oil
pink Himalayan salt or sea salt

1. Preheat the oven to 180°C/350°F/gas 4. Line two baking sheets with greaseproof paper.
2. Blitz the oats in a blender (I use the milling blade on the NutriBullet), but not too finely. A few chunks of oats are okay. Use 25g (¼ cup) of the oats to dust a work surface.
3. Mix the oats, bicarbonate of soda, a pinch of salt and the oregano together in a bowl, then stir in the olive oil and 125ml (½ cup) water to form a dough.
4. Roll out the dough on the oat-dusted surface to about 5mm thick.
5. Use a cutter or the top of a glass to cut into 6cm circles.
6. Place on the lined baking sheets and bake in the hot oven for 25 minutes, until crisp and golden, turning halfway.
7. Allow to cool and keep in an airtight container.

ENERGY BALLS – 3 WAYS

One of my favourite things to satisfy my cravings is energy balls. The main ingredients provide a healthy balance of fats, proteins and carbs, plus provide a punch of nutrients – exactly what you need to get you through a long day. Keep in the fridge and take a couple on-the-go as a snack each day.

SUPERFOOD

Makes 10

Ingredients

2 tbsp quinoa
80g (½ cup) unsalted raw almonds
60g (½ cup) raisins
90g (½ cup) medjool dates, pitted
30g (¼ cup) goji berries
1 tbsp chia seeds
1 tbsp maca powder

1. Place a saucepan on a medium-high heat. Add the quinoa, place the lid on and heat for about 2–3 minutes, shaking every few seconds. The quinoa will pop and slightly puff up.
2. Blend the almonds, raisins, dates and goji berries in a food processor until the mixture comes together. Add the remaining ingredients including the quinoa and roll into bite-size balls.

LEMON COCONUT BLISS

Makes 10

Ingredients

2 tbsp coconut oil
90g (1 cup) desiccated coconut
1 tbsp lemon zest
80g (½ cup) unsalted raw Brazil nuts
1 tsp vanilla powder or 1 teaspoon organic vanilla extract
2 tbsp maple syrup
3 tbsp lemon juice

1. Set aside the coconut oil, 3–4 tablespoons of the desiccated coconut and the lemon zest. Blend the remaining ingredients in a food processor until combined. Add the oil and pulse until combined.
2. Roll into bite-size balls and place in the fridge for 20 minutes.
3. Sprinkle the 3–4 tablespoons of desiccated coconut and the lemon zest onto a plate and roll the balls on the plate until fully covered.

SUPERGREEN

Makes 10

Ingredients

180g (1 cup) medjool dates, pitted
115g (¾ cup) unsalted raw cashew nuts
2 tsp spirulina
1 tsp wheatgrass
1 tbsp lime zest
1 tsp matcha powder

1. Blend all the ingredients except the matcha in a food processor until the mixture comes together.
2. Roll into bite-size balls and place in the fridge for 20 minutes.
3. Sprinkle the matcha powder onto a plate and roll the balls in it to coat.

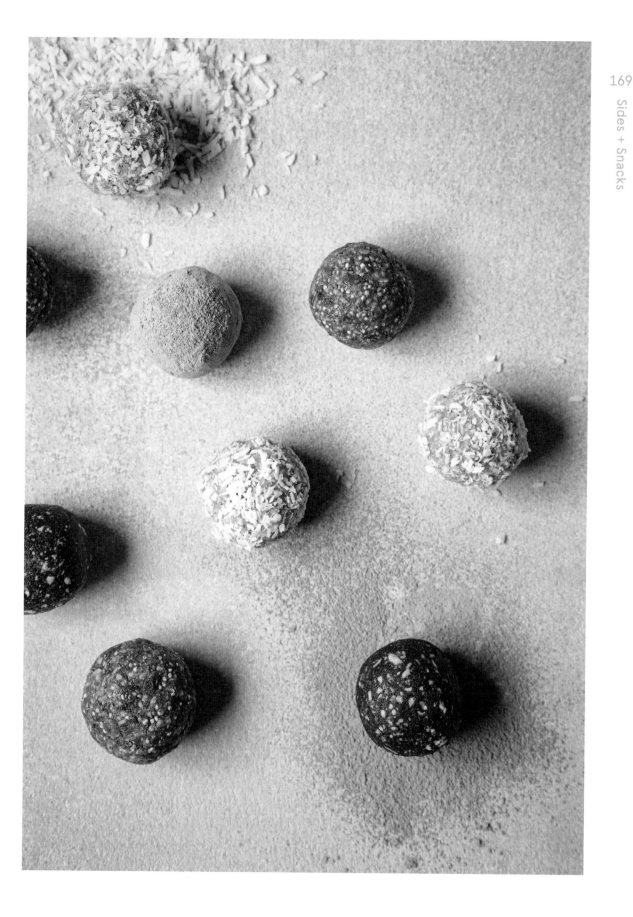

RAW FIG + BAOBAB BARS

Makes 12

As much as I love healthy nut and fruit bars from health food shops, there's just nothing quite like a homemade version, and it may be something that you haven't thought of making yourself before. I love the pop of the fig seeds and the sweetness from the sultanas in these.

Ingredients

320g (2 cups) unsulphured dried figs
310g (2 cups) unsalted raw cashew nuts
60g (½ cup) sultanas
30g (¼ cup) sunflower seeds
40g (¼ cup) linseeds
2 tbsp baobab powder

1. Trim the fig stalks, place the figs in a bowl, cover with water and set aside to soak for 1 hour.
2. Drain the figs and place all the ingredients apart from the baobab powder in a food processor or blender and blend. Add the baobab powder and blend until totally combined.
3. Bring the mixture together, then roll out into a large rectangle until about 1cm thick. It will be quite sticky.
4. Place in the freezer for 30 minutes to firm up, then neatly slice into bars roughly 3.5cm x 10cm and keep in an airtight container in the fridge.

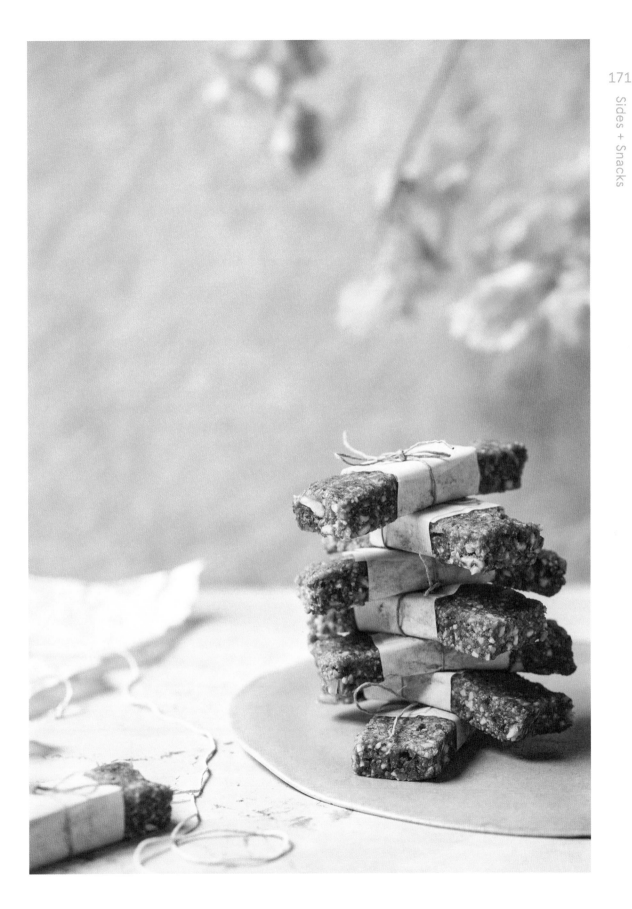

CHOCOLATE-COATED BANANA LOLLIES

Makes 6–8

These are another really quick, easy and delicious summer snack. The concept is simple but full of flavour. The lollipop sticks can be bought from most supermarkets and they look so pretty. The chocolate dip is homemade and needs only three ingredients.

Ingredients

2 large ripe bananas, peeled and cut into 1cm slices
2 tbsp almond butter
2 tbsp coconut oil
2 tbsp raw cacao powder
2 tbsp maple syrup
2 tbsp unsalted raw almonds

1. Spread each banana slice with almond butter and layer up 3-4 slices on each stick.
2. Place on a plate and repeat with the remaining banana slices and freeze for an hour.
3. To make the chocolate, heat the coconut oil in a small saucepan over a medium heat and remove from the heat just before it's totally melted. Whisk in the cacao powder and maple syrup, pour into a bowl and keep to one side.
4. Crush the almonds in a pestle and mortar until broken down into small chunks.
5. When the bananas have been freezing for at least an hour, remove and dip into the chocolate until totally covered. Immediately sprinkle the crushed almonds over the chocolate and place back in the freezer to set for about 30 minutes.

Tip ... To save yourself time making the homemade chocolate, feel free to melt dark chocolate instead.

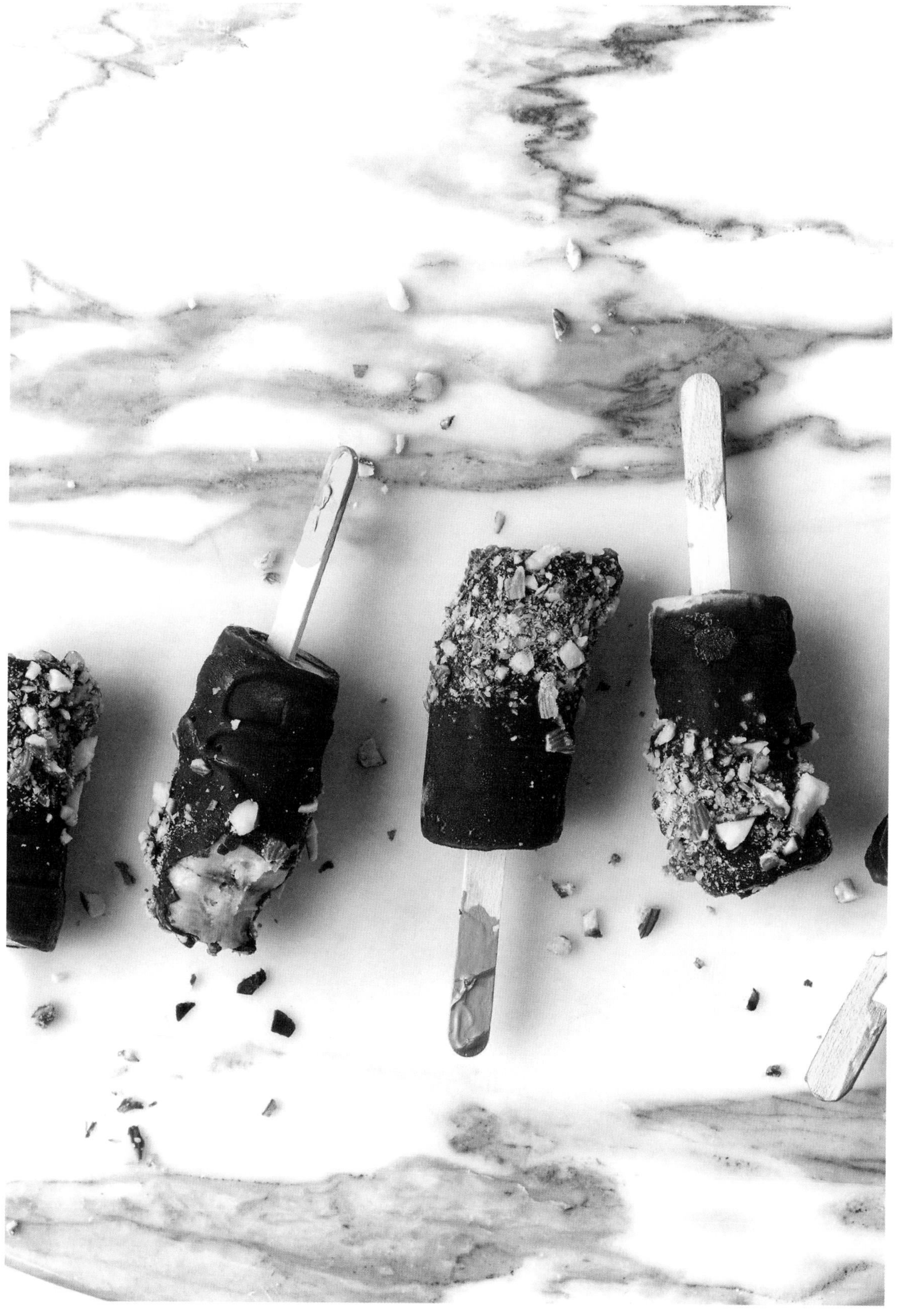

CHOCOLATE + FIG POPCORN BARS

Makes 10

For most people, watching a film at home just isn't the same without a bowl of popcorn, but after the saltiness of the popcorn you can often find yourself craving something sweet, too. So I've combined the two to make one incredible movie accompaniment.

Ingredients

- 6 dried figs (try to buy 100% natural figs without sulphur dioxide)
- ½ tsp coconut oil, plus extra for greasing
- 60g (½ cup) popcorn kernels
- 150g (1 cup) cacao butter
- 2½ tbsp raw cacao powder
- 3 tbsp pure maple syrup
- 60ml (¼ cup) almond butter
- 75g (½ cup) unsalted raw pistachios, chopped
- pink Himalayan salt or sea salt

1. Remove the stalks and place the figs in a bowl, then cover with water and leave to soak for at least 1 hour to soften.

2. Grease a 20cm square baking tin and line with greaseproof paper.

3. Heat the coconut oil in a large saucepan over a medium heat. Add the popcorn kernels and sprinkle over a pinch of salt. Give the saucepan a good shake and put the lid on.

4. It'll take a minute or so for the corn to start popping, and it should take 5–7 minutes for all the kernels to pop. Frequently shake the pan to make sure the kernels are being evenly cooked and to stop the pan from burning.

5. To make the chocolate, melt the cacao butter in a small saucepan over a low heat. Add the cacao powder and maple syrup to the pan and stir to combine.

6. Drain the figs that have been soaking and use the back of a fork to mash them into a paste. Stir them into the saucepan with the almond butter and half the chopped pistachios and remove from the heat.

7. Slowly transfer the popcorn into a large mixing bowl, discarding any kernels that haven't popped. Gradually pour the dark chocolate and fig mixture onto the popcorn, stirring as you go to make sure the popcorn is fully covered.

8. Pour the mixture into the lined baking tin and use the back of a spoon to spread it out evenly, scattering the remaining pistachios over the top. Gently compress the mixture with the spoon and place in the fridge for at least 2 hours to set, then slice into 10 bars.

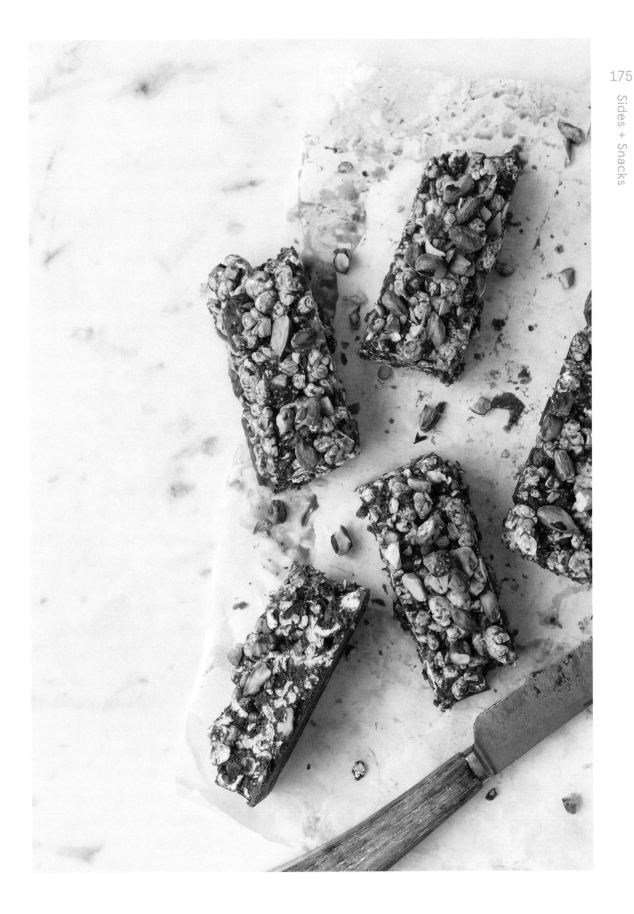

BLUEBERRY BURST DATES

Makes 10

I first tried cooked dates in Greece and I was surprised by how much they tasted of toffee. They were served as part of a savoury mezze and sprinkled with sea salt, but I've added a rich ginger flavour. The blueberry in the middle bursts when you bite into it, adding a sweet juicy taste.

Ingredients

10 medjool dates
10 blueberries
3 tbsp tahini
1½ tsp ground ginger
pink Himalayan salt or sea salt

1. Preheat the oven to 170°C/325°F/gas 3. Line a baking sheet with greaseproof paper.
2. Slice the dates down one side lengthways, remove the pit and open them out like a book. Sprinkle over a small amount of salt and place a blueberry in the middle of each date.
3. Place on the baking sheet and bake in the hot oven for 15 minutes, checking about halfway through. Allow to cool until warm.
4. Make the filling by mixing the tahini with the ginger and spooning about a teaspoon into each date.

Tip ... If you don't have tahini, try almond butter instead.

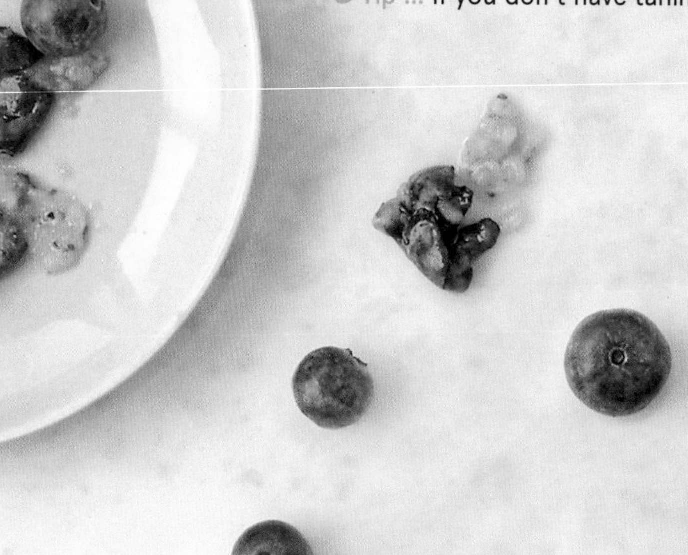

BOMBAY POPCORN

Serves 4

Popcorn is a wonderful snack alternative to crisps that doesn't have all the additives. Although light, it keeps you feeling full and you can experiment with many different flavours. One of my favourite combinations is this Indian-inspired spice mix. Try making this on your next film night in!

Ingredients

1 tsp coconut oil
110g (½ cup) popcorn kernels
¼ tsp each of ground cumin, coriander, turmeric and ground ginger or 1 tsp curry powder
pink Himalayan salt or sea salt and freshly ground black pepper

1. Heat the coconut oil in a large lidded saucepan over a medium-high heat.
2. Once melted, add the popcorn kernels with the spices and a pinch of salt and pepper, then shake the pan to make sure all the kernels are coated.
3. Place the lid on, turn the heat down to medium and wait for the kernels to start to pop, shaking the pan occasionally.
4. When the popcorn has finished popping, remove from the heat and tip into a large bowl, discarding any unpopped kernels.

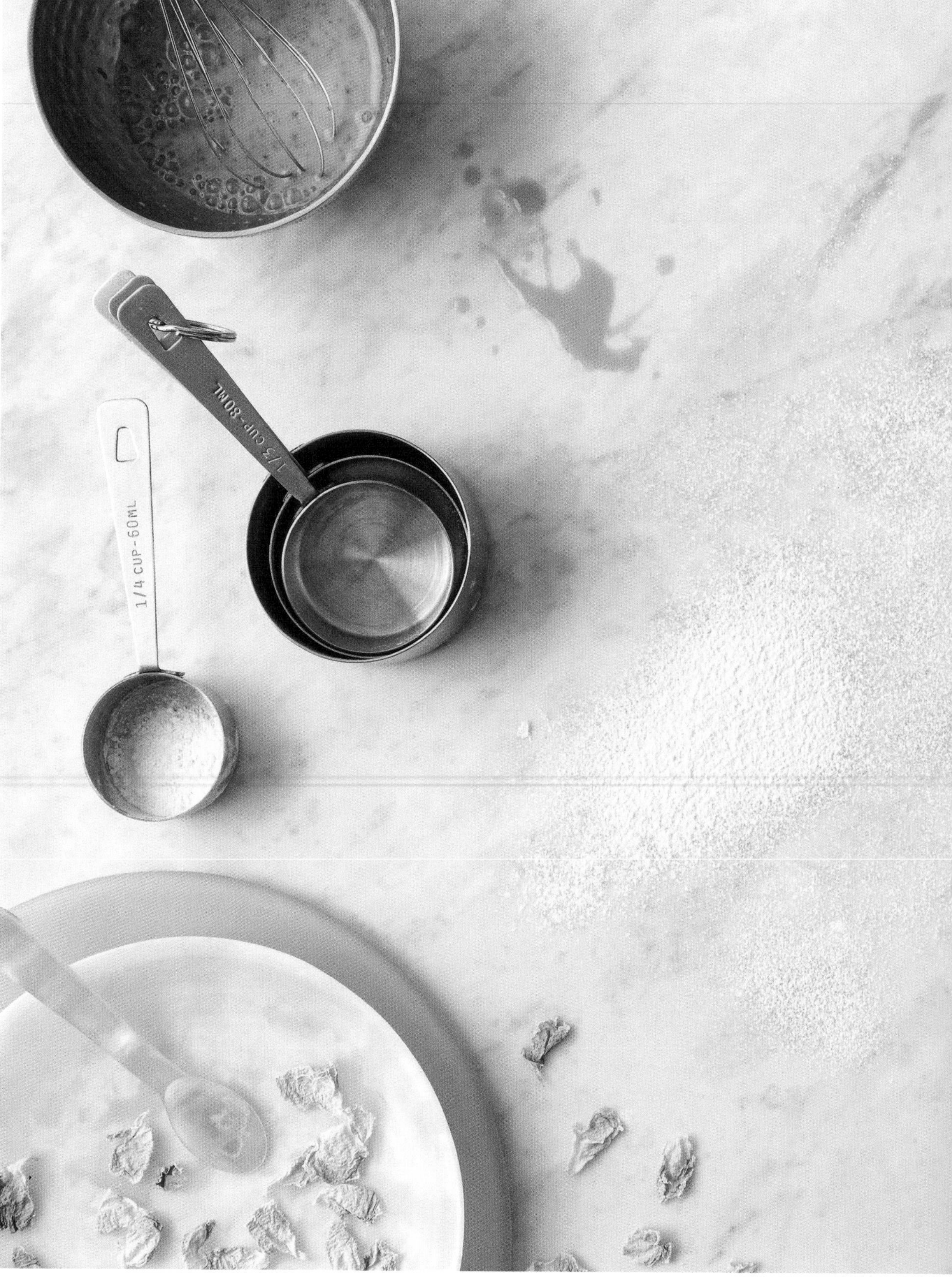
1/3 CUP-80ML
1/4 CUP-60ML

Dessert

Ø5

AFTER-DINNER TRUFFLES

Makes 10

A few years ago if you'd told me I could eat healthier truffles I would have laughed, but then I discovered dates! Dates are deliciously sweet and when combined with molasses they provide a rich truffle flavour. These are perfect for an evening treat when I'm watching my favourite TV programme.

Ingredients

200g (1 cup) medjool dates, pitted
125g (½ cup) unsalted peanut butter
50g (½ cup) rolled oats
1 tsp blackstrap molasses
a pinch of Himalayan pink salt or sea salt
2 tbsp raw cacao powder, to coat

1. Blend all the ingredients except the cacao powder in a food processor until the mixture sticks together.
2. Roll into 10 bite-size balls and place in the fridge for 20 minutes to cool.
3. Sprinkle the cacao powder onto a plate and roll each of the balls on the plate twice to make sure they're fully coated. Keep refrigerated in an airtight container.

Tip ... For a milder flavour, almond butter works really well in this recipe instead of peanut butter.

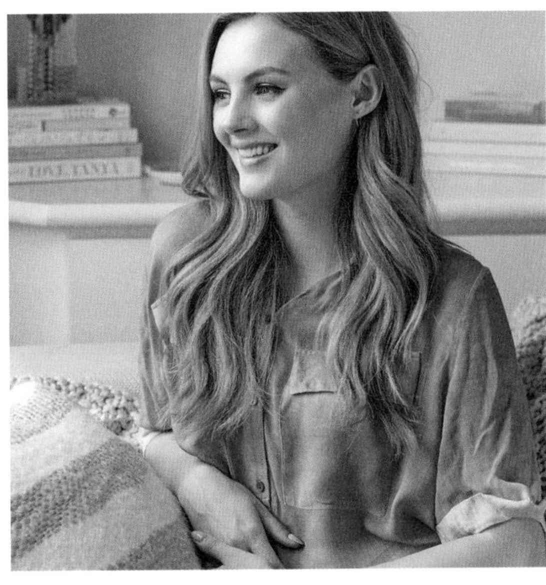

RASPBERRY + LEMON RIPPLE CHEESECAKE

Serves 10

This is a beautiful dessert and one I love to make when I want to impress the family. The mixture brings together two of my favourite colours and flavours: pink raspberry and yellow lemon. To recreate a biscuit base I use pistachios, and almonds for their crunchy texture.

Ingredients

base

- 180g (1 cup) medjool dates, pitted
- 40g (¼ cup) unsalted raw pistachios
- 115g (¾ cup) unsalted raw almonds

filling

- 1 lemon
- 1 x 400g tin coconut milk, refrigerated
- 310g (2 cups) unsalted raw cashew nuts, soaked overnight
- 60ml (¼ cup) coconut nectar, agave nectar or honey
- 60ml (¼ cup) coconut oil
- seeds of 1 vanilla pod or 1 tsp organic vanilla extract
- 185g (1¼ cups) raspberries

- 2 tbsp pistachios, chopped, to serve
- 2 tbsp edible rose petals (optional), to serve

1. Blend all the base ingredients together in a food processor until combined. Tip the mixture into a 20cm loose-bottomed cake tin and press down firmly with the back of a wooden spoon. Place in the freezer while you make the filling.

2. Zest the lemon and keep to one side, then squeeze the juice into a food processor or blender. Scoop out the solid coconut cream that has risen to the top of the tin of coconut milk (this should be around 150g) and add to the blender with a couple of tablespoons of the milk. Drain the cashews and add with the remaining filling ingredients, except the raspberries, and blend until smooth and creamy (if you have a NutriBullet, use this here to blend in batches – it will create a lovely smooth texture).

3. Set aside 60ml (¼ cup) of the mixture. Stir 90g (¾ cup) of the raspberries and half the lemon zest into the remaining cheesecake mixture. Remove the base from the freezer and pour over half the cheesecake mixture.

4. Blend the reserved 60ml (¼ cup) of the cheesecake mixture with the remaining raspberries until totally smooth. Add half this mixture, a tablespoon at a time, to the top of the cheesecake, gently swirling with a chopstick or the end of a spoon to create a ripple effect.

5. Pour over the remaining plain cheesecake mixture and smooth down. Again, add a tablespoon at a time of the remaining raspberry cheesecake mixture and create ripple effects. Gently shake the tin to smooth the top.

6. Mix the chopped pistachios with the rose petals, if using, and scatter on top of the cheesecake. Sprinkle the remaining lemon zest over the top and freeze for at least 4 hours, preferably overnight.
7. Take the cheesecake out of the freezer 30 minutes before serving, to thaw, or transfer to the fridge for about an hour and a half.

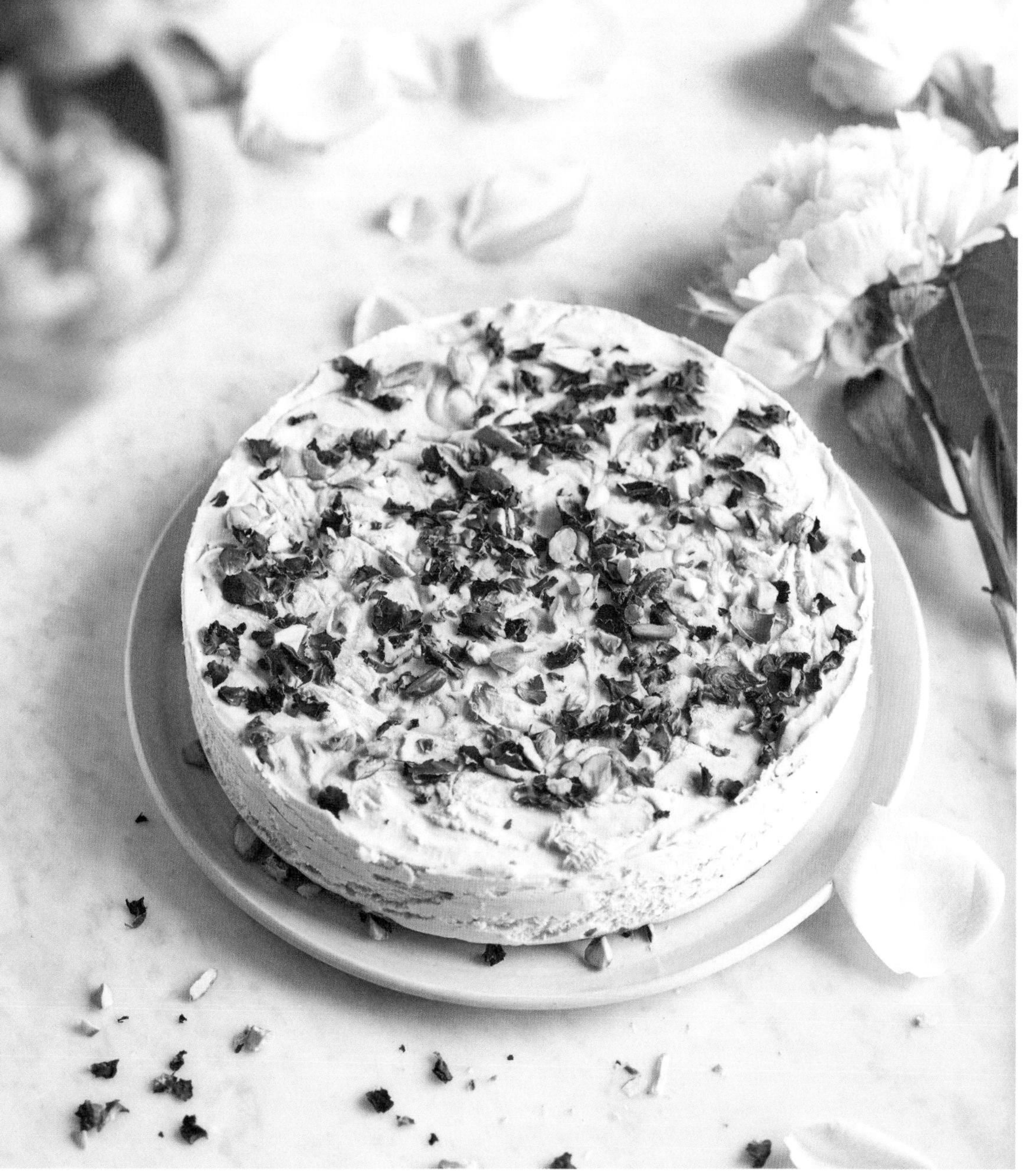

ORANGE + BASIL TART

Serves 10

I love to end a dinner party with this tart; it's sophisticated, light and pleasing on the palate. The secret ingredient is steamed, blended butternut squash, which makes a beautifully smooth and creamy filling. Don't be put off by vegetables in desserts, it's great to experiment and when you get it right it's so rewarding.

Ingredients

filling
½ butternut squash, peeled and chopped
1 x 400g tin of coconut milk, refrigerated
75ml (⅓ cup) maple syrup
1 tsp organic vanilla extract
zest of 1 orange, juice of ½
8–10 fresh basil leaves

crust
150g (1½ cups) ground almonds
135g (¾ cup) medjool dates, pitted
1½ tbsp raw cacao powder
zest of 2 small oranges

topping
1 tbsp orange zest
a few fresh baby basil leaves

1. Place the squash in a lidded steamer basket. Steam for 15–20 minutes over a medium saucepan of simmering water until soft. Remove from the heat and allow to cool (to make this quicker, run it under cold water).
2. Now make the crust. Use a food processor to mix all the ingredients together until the mixture is sticky and holds together.
3. Press the mixture into a circular 20cm fluted tart tin, making sure you press the crust right into the ridges, then keep in the fridge while you make the filling.
4. Use a food processor or a hand whisk to blend the steamed butternut squash until smooth. You will need 1 cup of this butternut squash purée, so if there's any leftover, save the rest for lunch!
5. Scoop out the solid coconut cream that has risen to the top of the tin of coconut milk (this should be around 150g), place in the food processor with the remaining ingredients and blend until smooth.
6. Pour into the cooled crust and place in the fridge for a few hours to set, preferably overnight.
7. Serve soon after removing from the fridge, scattered with a grating of orange zest and a few baby basil leaves.

Tip ... Refrigerating coconut milk in the can encourages the solids to separate from the liquid and rise to the top. These solids work perfectly in recipes like this to give a lovely creamy consistency.

APPLE + APRICOT CRUMBLE

Serves 4–6

My mum used to make a wonderful rhubarb crumble when I was younger; it is so nostalgic so I wanted to create my own version. I've paired apple and apricot; one of my favourite flavour combinations. My twist here is using oats, which are much more filling. Bring to the centre of the table and let everyone dig in!

Ingredients

4 Bramley apples
5 tbsp coconut sugar
1 tsp ground cinnamon
a pinch of ground nutmeg
a pinch of ground cloves
½ tsp ground ginger
90g (½ cup) unsulphured dried apricots, quartered
200g (1⅓ cups) unsalted raw almonds
125g (1¼ cups) rolled oats
a pinch of pink Himalayan salt or sea salt
75ml (⅓ cup) coconut oil

1. Preheat the oven to 180°C/350°F/gas 4.
2. Peel and core the apples and chop into rough 2cm chunks. Place in a medium saucepan over a medium-low heat and add enough water to just cover the base of the pan. Cover the pan with a lid.
3. Simmer for 7 minutes over a medium heat until softened and starting to break down, stirring occasionally, then remove from the heat.
4. Stir in 2 tablespoons of the sugar, the spices and apricots and keep to one side while you make the crumble.
5. In a small saucepan make a caramel by heating the remaining coconut sugar with 60ml (¼ cup) water over a medium heat. Keep stirring and remove from the heat when a sticky, caramel consistency has formed.
6. Whizz 50g (½ cup) of the almonds in a food processor until fine. Then add the remaining almonds and 50g (½ cup) of the oats and whizz until a crumbly consistency has formed. Tip into a large bowl and combine with the remaining whole oats, caramel and a pinch of salt.
7. Melt the coconut oil in a small saucepan over a low heat, add to the bowl and stir to combine.
8. Pour the stewed apple into a 20cm square ovenproof baking dish, add the crumble on top and bake in the hot oven for 30 minutes.

Serving ideas ...

For a real treat, try this with my Pecan ice cream (see page 186).

PECAN ICE CREAM WITH SALTED CARAMEL SAUCE

Serves 4

We all get those moments when we crave ice cream, and you'd never guess this is made from plant-based ingredients. One of my favourite flavours is salted caramel pecan, and when dates are blended with salt you get that same rich caramel flavour, without the refined sugar.

Ingredients

pecan ice cream

- seeds of 1 vanilla pod or 1 tsp vanilla powder
- 50g (½ cup) unsalted raw pecan nuts
- 5 medjool dates, pitted
- 250ml (1 cup) unsweetened almond milk
- 1 x 400g tin coconut milk
- 1 tbsp almond butter
- a pinch of pink Himalayan salt or sea salt

salted caramel sauce

- 5 medjool dates, pitted and soaked
- 125ml (½ cup) unsweetened almond milk
- a pinch of pink Himalayan salt or sea salt

- a handful of unsalted raw pecan nuts, chopped, to serve

1. To make the pecan ice cream, start by removing the seeds from the vanilla pod. Slice down one side and gently open up the pod and use the knife or a teaspoon to scrape out the seeds.

2. Take half of the seeds or half of the vanilla powder and blitz with half the pecans and the remaining ingredients in a blender for a couple of minutes until smooth.

3. Pour into a large plastic container, crumble in the remaining pecans and stir.

4. Freeze for 3 hours, stirring every 30 minutes, if you can.

5. To make the salted caramel sauce, drain the dates and blend with the almond milk and remaining vanilla pod seeds or powder in a blender until totally smooth. Stir in the sea salt and keep in the fridge until you need it later.

6. After 3 hours of freezing, remove the ice cream from the freezer and use an electric whisk to whizz up the mixture so that it's extra smooth and creamy, then place back in the freezer for another hour. This is optional, so don't worry if you skip this step.

7. After the ice cream has been freezing for 4 hours, gently swirl in two thirds of the caramel sauce to make a ripple effect and place back in the freezer overnight (or for at least another 2 hours).

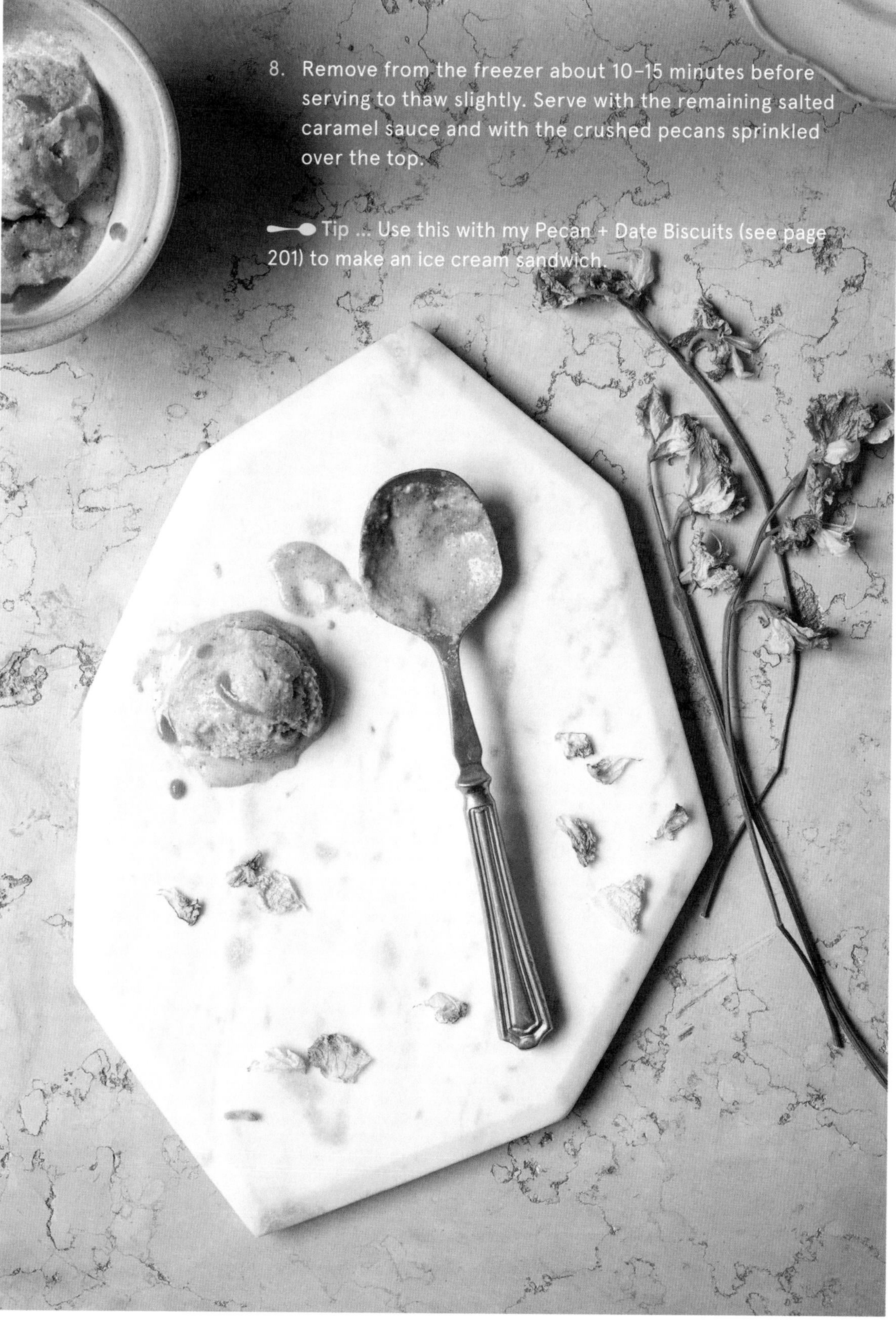

8. Remove from the freezer about 10–15 minutes before serving to thaw slightly. Serve with the remaining salted caramel sauce and with the crushed pecans sprinkled over the top.

Tip ... Use this with my Pecan + Date Biscuits (see page 201) to make an ice cream sandwich.

BANANA MOCHA ICE CREAM CUPS

Makes 8

I don't have coffee too often, but once in a while it's a wonderful hit of energy and a great addition to a dessert. These cream cups only have a subtle hint of coffee, so even if you don't like it it's a nice way to introduce it to your palate.

Ingredients

1 tbsp instant coffee
3 ripe bananas, peeled, sliced and frozen
1 tsp organic vanilla extract
3 tbsp raw cacao powder
125ml (½ cup) tinned coconut milk
2–3 tbsp maple syrup
dark chocolate, to serve
coffee beans, to serve

1. Dissolve the instant coffee with 1 tablespoon boiling water and set aside to cool slightly.
2. Place the frozen bananas in a food processor (check your food processor works with ice) and pulse until broken down, then whizz on a high speed until thickened and creamy.
3. Add the coffee, vanilla extract, cacao powder, coconut milk and maple syrup and pulse again until combined, stopping every now and again to scrape the sides of the food processor to make sure everything is combined.
4. Spoon into silicone cupcake cases and place in the freezer for about 2 hours.
5. Remove from the freezer 15 minutes before serving to soften. Grate dark chocolate over the top and place a coffee bean on each cup.

Tip ... This recipe makes 8, so it's the perfect make-ahead dessert for large dinner parties.

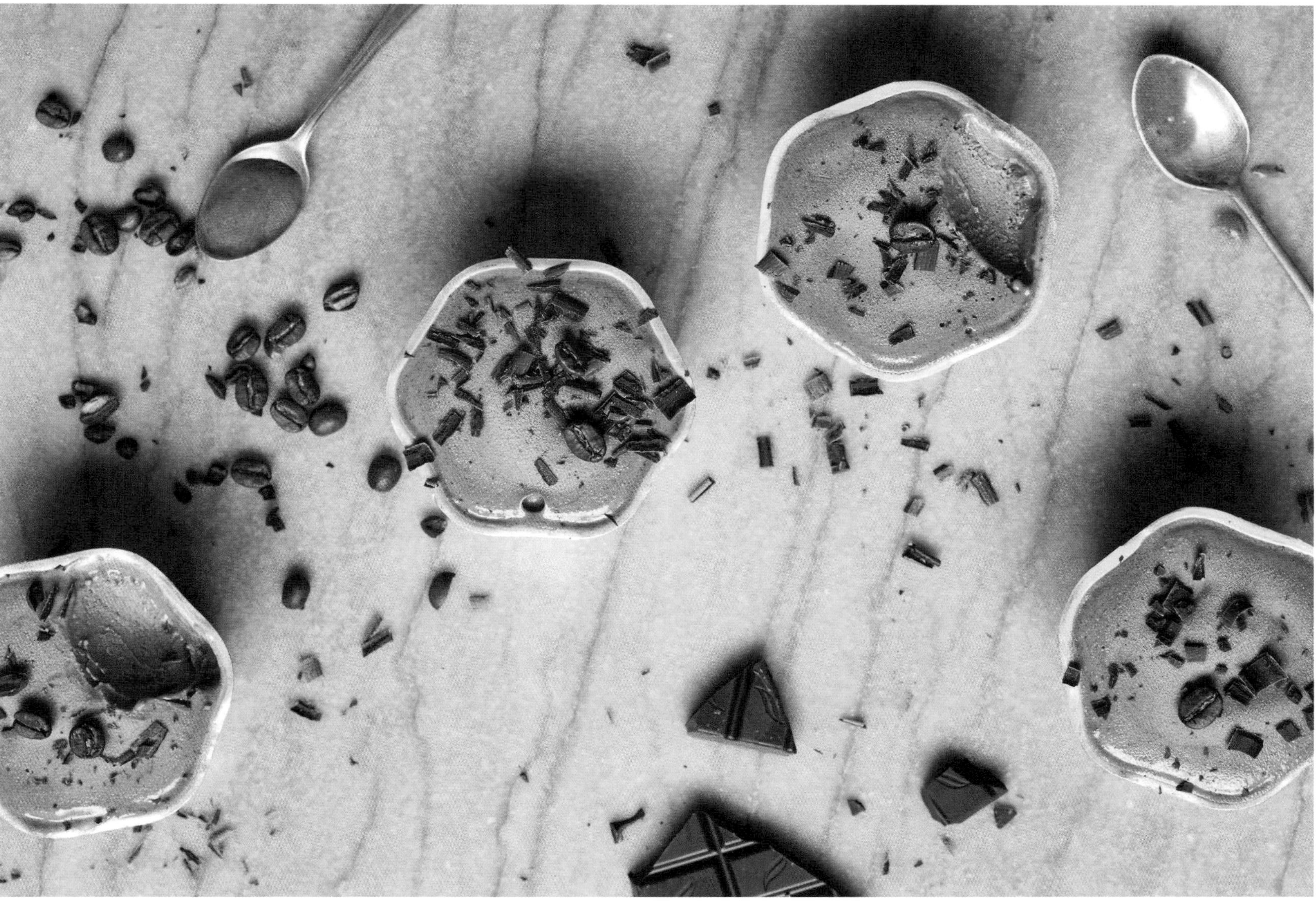

CHOCOLATE COOKIE DOUGH ICE CREAM

Serves 4

One of the best things about bananas when they are frozen and blended is that you get the consistency and creaminess of ice cream. This is inspired by one of my old favourites while I was at university, cookie dough ice cream. Instead of vanilla I wanted to make this chocolate flavoured by adding cacao powder. This is great for a night in with friends and a good film.

Ingredients

chocolate ice cream

6 frozen ripe bananas, peeled
1 ½ tsp organic vanilla extract
2 tbsp raw cacao powder
2 tbsp maple syrup (optional)

cookie dough pieces

25g (¼ cup) rolled oats
½ tbsp coconut oil
1 tbsp maple syrup
½ tbsp almond butter
25g (¼ cup) ground almonds
1 tbsp dark chocolate chips

a handful of raspberries, to serve

1. Grind the oats to a flour in a food processor.
2. Gently heat the coconut oil in a saucepan over a low heat until melted. Remove from the heat, add the maple syrup and almond butter and stir to combine.
3. In a large bowl, mix together the ground almonds and oat flour. Stir in the coconut oil mixture. Allow to cool slightly before adding the dark chocolate chips.
4. Roll into small balls (use about ½ teaspoon of mixture for each) and pinch the sides to make small cubes. Freeze for about 10-15 minutes.
5. Meanwhile, make the ice cream. Blend the frozen bananas with the vanilla extract, cacao powder and maple syrup, if using, in a blender that works with ice until creamy and smooth.
6. Pour into two bowls and top with 5 cookie dough pieces each and some raspberries.

Tip ... If you have cookie dough left over, keep them in the fridge in an airtight container and eat as treats.

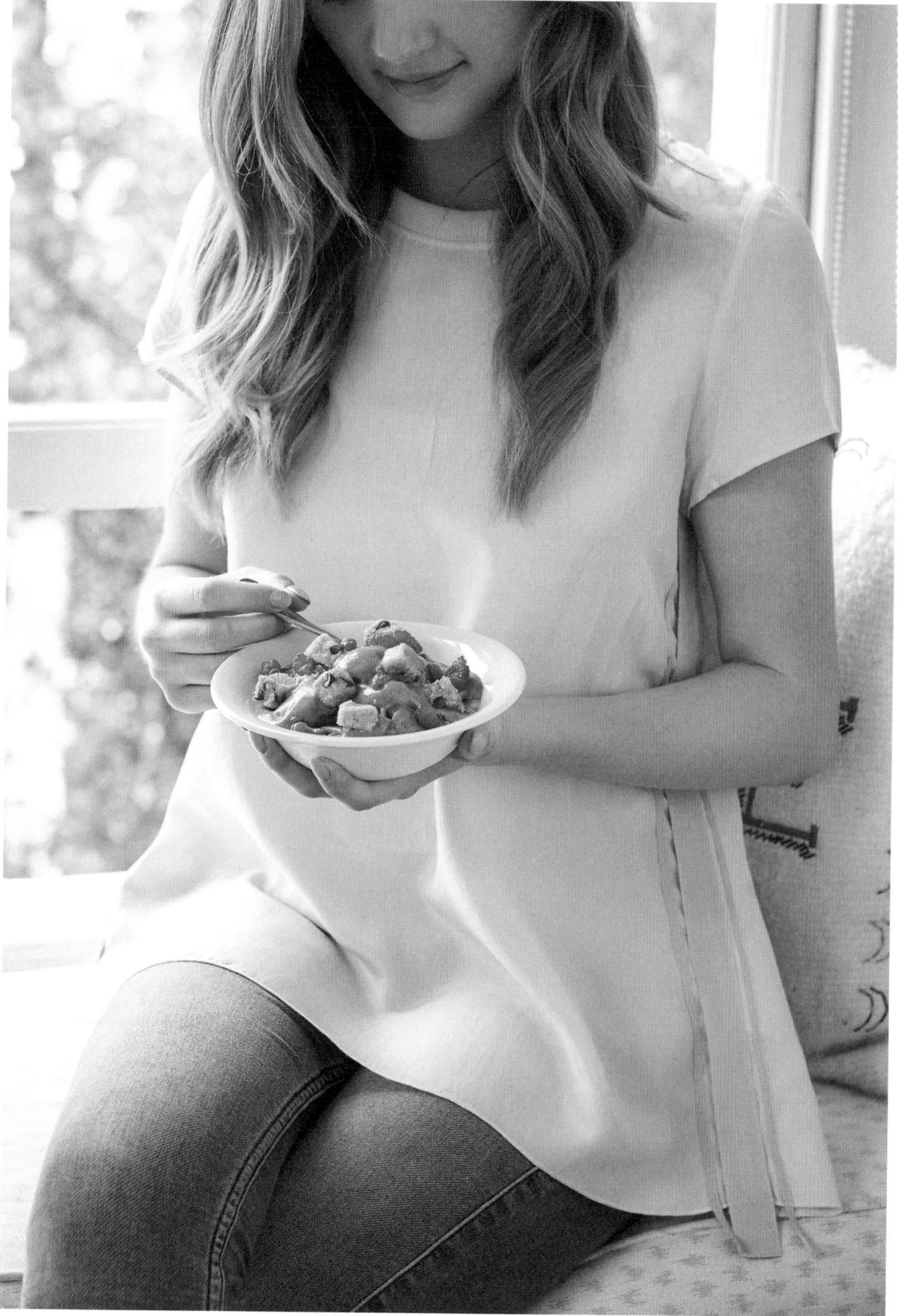

EASY WATERMELON SORBET

Serves 4

When I think about cooling down in the summer, there is something about watermelon and mint when paired together that is so refreshing. Watermelon is great for hydration and mint is really soothing, making the perfect combination. I love this after a meal or as an afternoon snack on a hot day.

Ingredients

½ watermelon
1 ripe banana, peeled
250ml (1 cup) fresh orange juice or water
a handful of fresh mint leaves
4 lemon wedges

1. Deseed the watermelon and cut the flesh into about 2cm thick chunks. Freeze for 5 hours or overnight, laying the chunks flat on a tray or plate so they don't stick together.
2. Once frozen, place in a blender that works with ice with the banana, juice or water and blend until almost smooth. Just before it is totally blended, add the mint leaves and blend until totally smooth.
3. Scoop into bowls and serve with a wedge of lemon to squeeze over the top.

Tip ... These ingredients also make a nice smoothie; just whizz together instead of freezing.

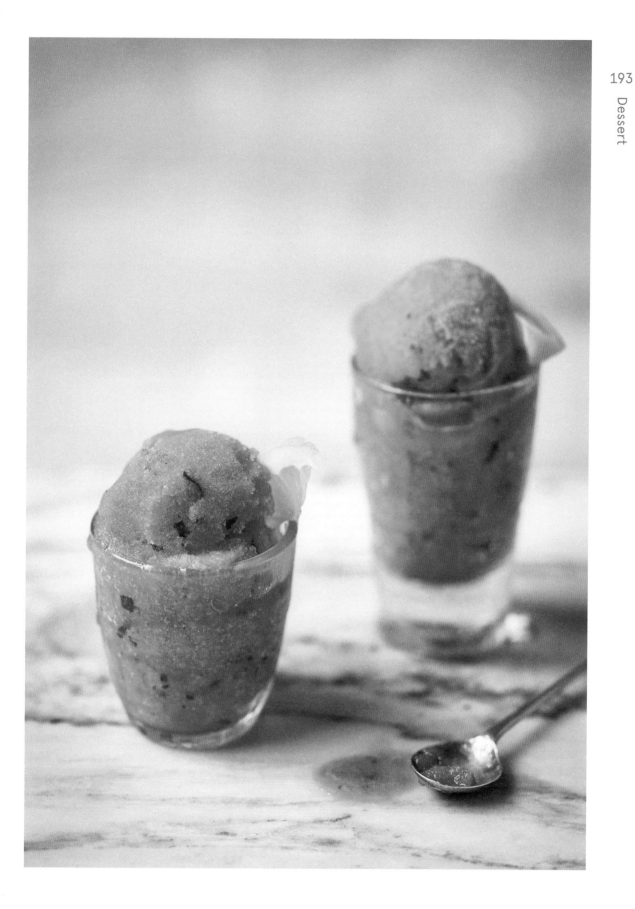

ICE LOLLIES – 3 WAYS

I love making ice lollies in the summer; they are super refreshing and a tasty way to cool down. These are 100% fruit and an easy dessert for a BBQ or picnic. When I know my younger cousins are coming I always make a big batch for the freezer – they particularly love the mango.

MANGO + COCONUT

Makes 2

Ingredients

1 lime
½ mango, peeled and stoned
1 tbsp desiccated coconut

1. Zest the lime and keep to one side.
2. Roughly chop the mango and place in a blender with the lime juice and 80ml (⅓ cup) water. Whizz until smooth, then stir in the desiccated coconut and the lime zest.
3. Pour into two lolly moulds and freeze for at least 5 hours, until solid.

APPLE COOLER

Makes 2

Ingredients

¼ cucumber, peeled
3 fresh mint leaves
1 green apple, peeled

1. Finely chop the cucumber and mint leaves, then keep to one side and roughly chop the remaining cucumber. Core and roughly chop the apple.
1. Place the apple and cucumber chunks into a blender with 60ml (¼ cup) water. Whizz until smooth, then stir in the finely chopped mint and cucumber.
2. Pour into two lolly moulds and freeze for at least 5 hours, until solid.

SUMMER BERRY

Makes 2

Ingredients

30g (¼ cup) raspberries, plus 3 extra
40g (¼ cup) blueberries, plus 3 extra

1. Place the berries in a blender with 80ml (⅓ cup) water and whizz until smooth.
2. Drop the extra berries into two lolly moulds, pour in the blended mixture and freeze for at least 5 hours, until solid.

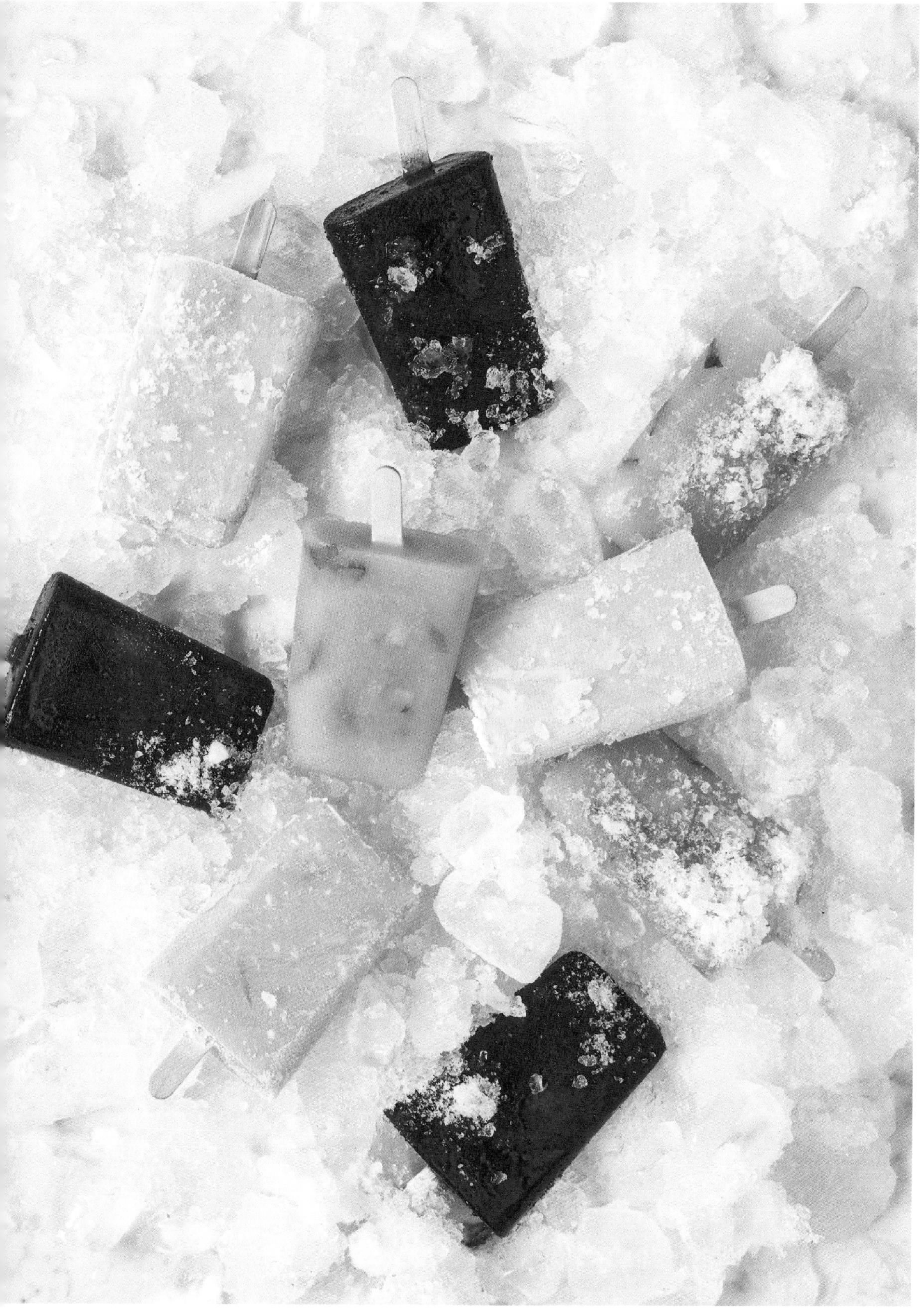

BALINESE BLACK RICE PUDDING WITH MANGO

Serves 2

In Bali a traditional breakfast dish is a black rice pudding usually cooked by the grandmothers early in the morning. When I tried this for the first time I fell in love. I wanted to make it into a dessert because it's a bit too sweet for me for breakfast, but I love the simple flavour combination.

Ingredients

100g (½ cup) black rice
1 vanilla pod
4 tbsp tinned coconut milk
2 tbsp coconut nectar or palm sugar
a pinch of pink Himalayan salt or sea salt

toppings
2 tbsp coconut flakes
½ mango, peeled, stoned and diced
2 tbsp tinned coconut milk
coconut nectar (optional)

1. Place the rice in a sieve and rinse thoroughly under cold running water, then soak in a bowl of water for at least 1 hour, or overnight if possible. This will make the rice softer.

2. Drain and add to a saucepan with 250ml (1 cup) water. Bring to the boil with a pinch of salt, then turn the heat down to low and simmer for 1 hour, adding more water if it gets too dry and stirring every now and again.

3. Once cooked, drain and return the rice to the pan. Slice down the length of the vanilla pod, scrape out the seeds and stir into the cooked rice with the coconut milk and the coconut nectar or sugar.

4. Toast the coconut flakes in a dry frying pan over a medium-high heat for a couple of minutes until golden, stirring frequently, to prevent burning.

5. Top the rice with the mango, a drizzle of coconut milk and a drizzle of coconut nectar, if you like. Scatter the toasted coconut over the top and dig in.

Tip ... If you can't get hold of a vanilla pod use a teaspoon of vanilla extract.

CHOCOLATE + BANANA CHIA PUDDING

Serves 2

A pudding can seem mega indulgent, but when it's full of the good stuff like avocado and banana you're hitting the spot on flavour and nutrition. Adding the chia seeds brings a new dimension to the dish – they are hydrating and packed with nutritional value for your brain and skin.

Ingredients

2 tbsp chia seeds
1 ripe banana, peeled
3 medjool dates, pitted
½ ripe avocado, peeled and stoned
2 tbsp raw cacao powder
125ml (½ cup) unsweetened almond milk

1. Soak the chia seeds with 6 tablespoons water in a bowl and refrigerate for about 20 minutes.
2. Put all the ingredients apart from the soaked chia seeds into a blender and whizz until smooth and the dates have broken up.
3. Stir in the soaked chia seeds and pour the mixture into two bowls or glasses. Top with your choice of toppings and tuck in.

Topping ideas ...

A handful of fresh or frozen raspberries
Granola (see page 46)
A handful of pumpkin seeds
A dusting of cacao powder

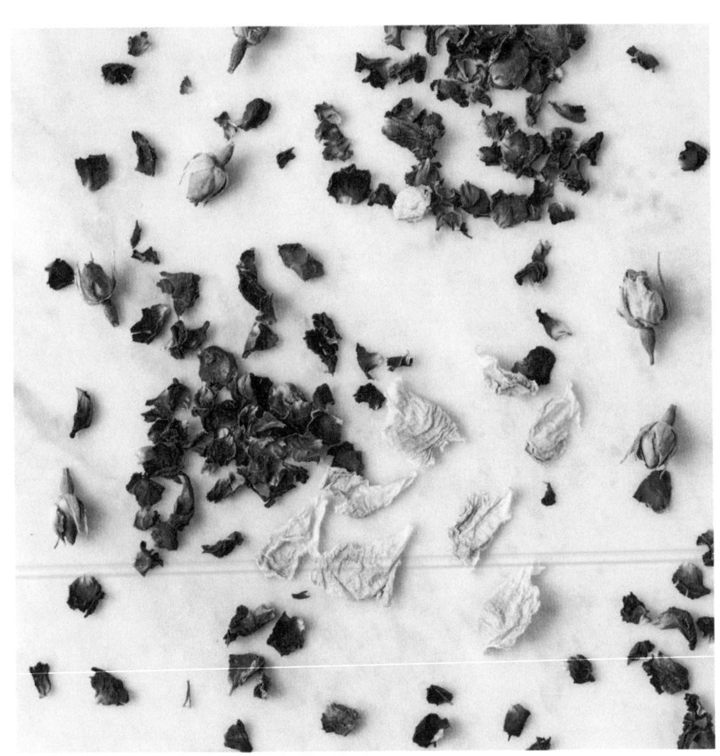

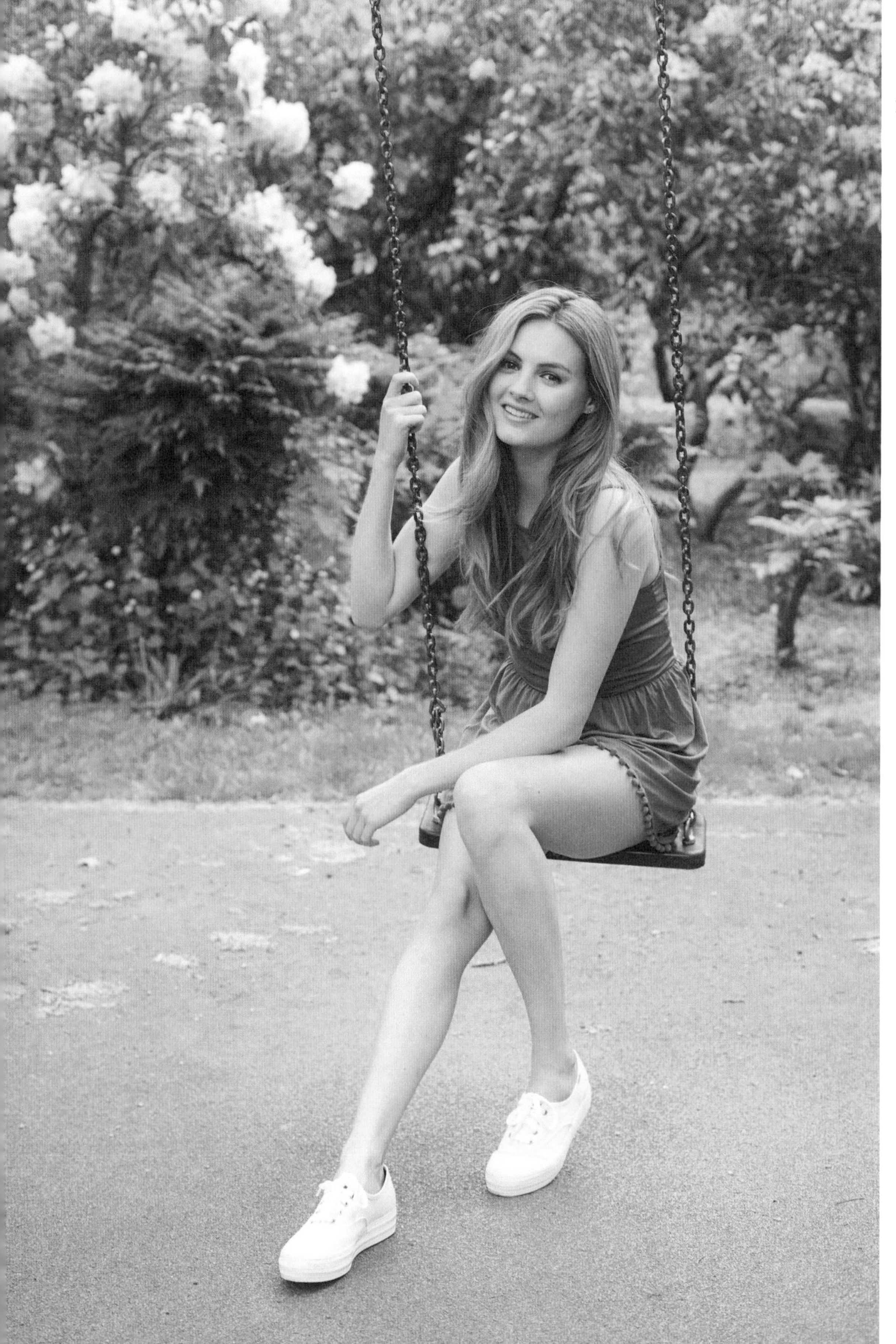

BANANA + CHOC CHIP MUFFINS

Makes 8

I love straight-out-of-the-oven muffins. These are a nice treat to take with you on the go in between meetings or to bake for the family. If you're working from home and you crave an afternoon treat, they can be whipped up really quickly, with no need to cave in to shop-bought biscuits!

Ingredients

dry ingredients

200g (1½ cups) spelt flour
1 tsp baking powder
3 tbsp coconut sugar
½ tsp vanilla powder
50g (¼ cup) dark chocolate chips (dairy-free)

wet ingredients

3 heaped tbsp coconut oil
3 ripe bananas, peeled
80ml (⅓ cup) unsweetened almond milk

1. Preheat the oven to 180°C/350°F/gas 4. Line a muffin tin with paper muffin cases.
2. In a large bowl, mix together all the dry ingredients apart from the chocolate chips.
3. Melt the coconut oil in a small saucepan over a low heat. Mash the bananas with a fork and mix together with the melted coconut oil and almond milk. Tip into the bowl of dry ingredients and stir in the chocolate chips.
4. Spoon the mixture evenly into eight muffin cases and bake in the hot oven for 25–30 minutes until a knife inserted comes out clean. Allow to cool in the tin for 5 minutes, then transfer to a wire rack to cool completely.

Tip ... If your bananas aren't quite ripe, place them in a brown paper bag with an apple or pear for a few hours. I find this helps them to ripen quicker.

PECAN + DATE BISCUITS

Makes 18

Rather than spending hours looking for presents on the high street or online, why not bring these to your next birthday party or event instead? I love to wrap these in pretty brown paper and some string. They look great and will keep for a few days after the party.

Ingredients

2 tbsp milled flaxseed
200g (2 cups) rolled oats
125g (1 cup) unsalted raw pecan nuts, finely chopped
½ tsp ground cinnamon
½ tsp bicarbonate of soda
a pinch of pink Himalayan salt or sea salt
180g (1 cup) medjool dates, preferably soaked overnight
½ tsp organic vanilla extract

1. Preheat the oven to 170°C/325°F/gas 3. Line two baking sheets with greaseproof paper.
2. Mix the flaxseed with 3 tablespoons water and keep to one side to thicken for at least 10 minutes.
3. Grind half the oats to a flour in a food processor and mix with the whole oats, chopped pecan nuts, cinnamon, bicarbonate of soda and a pinch of salt.
4. If soaking the dates, reserve half of the soaking water and drain the rest. Place the dates, reserved water and vanilla extract in a food processor and blend until smooth, then stir in the flaxseed mixture, which should have thickened by now.
5. In a large bowl combine the dry ingredients in the date mixture.
6. Scoop a heaped tablespoon of the mixture onto the lined baking tray. Use your fingers to press down to create a biscuit shape.
7. Repeat until all the mixture has been used. Bake in the hot oven for 10–12 minutes, then remove from the oven.
8. Allow to cool before removing the biscuits from the baking paper and store in an airtight container.

Tip ... Soaking the dates softens them, and using the soaking water in the recipe adds delicious flavour. Simply place the dates in a bowl of water overnight.

ORANGE SPICED BISCUITS

Makes 18

This is a lovely festive treat. It has all the typical ingredients that you get in Christmas pudding in a light delicious cookie. There is something about the smell of oranges and cinnamon that reminds me so much of Christmas, while ground almonds give it a nutty texture and taste.

Ingredients

dry ingredients

- 150g (1½ cups) ground almonds
- 200g (1½ cups) spelt flour
- 1 tsp bicarbonate of soda
- 1 tsp ground cinnamon
- ½ tsp ground ginger
- ¼ tsp ground nutmeg
- a pinch of ground cloves
- 115g (½ cup) coconut sugar

wet ingredients

- 125ml (½ cup) coconut oil
- 1 orange
- 1 tbsp black strap molasses
- 1 tsp apple cider vinegar

1. Preheat the oven to 190°C/375°F/gas 5. Line two baking sheets with greaseproof paper.
2. Mix the dry ingredients except the coconut sugar together in a large bowl and set aside.
3. Gently heat the coconut oil in a small saucepan over a low heat until just melted. Remove from the heat and beat with the coconut sugar by hand or with an electric whisk until combined.
4. Zest the orange and set aside. In a large bowl, squeeze in the juice from the orange and pour in the remaining wet ingredients, with the combined coconut sugar and melted coconut oil.
5. Use an electric hand whisk to mix on a high speed for about 1 minute.
6. Gently fold in the dry ingredients with the orange zest, adding one half at a time, until combined.
7. Divide the mixture into 18 balls and place them on the baking sheets. Flatten them into 5cm rounds and bake in the hot oven for 10-12 minutes until golden.

Tip ... To make this nut-free, swap the ground almonds for ground oats.

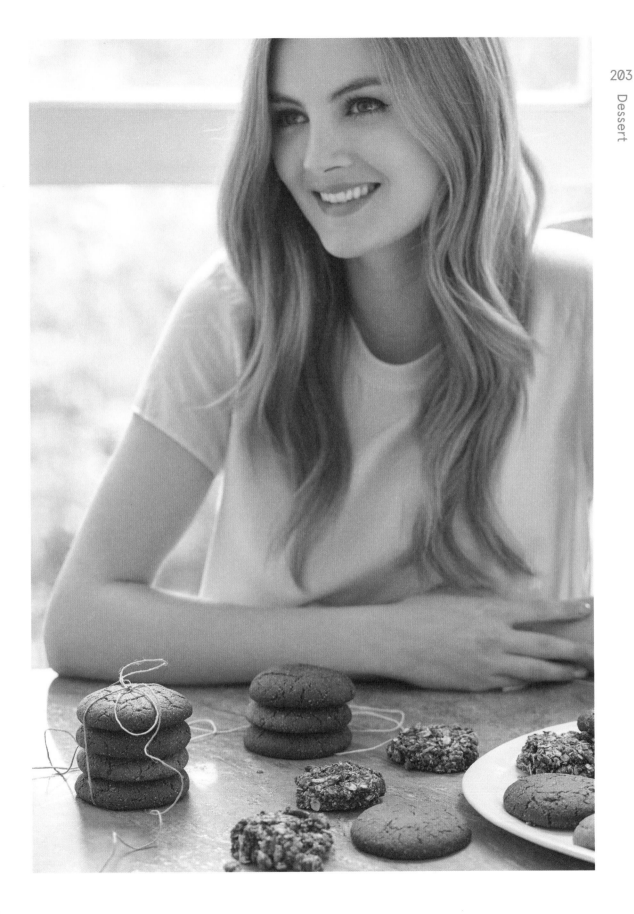

JAMMY DODGERS

Makes 25

I know so many people will identify with my school-day memories of opening my lunch box and finding a jammy dodger inside. These are great to have in the biscuit tin if someone pops in unexpectedly, as they probably won't have had one in years. But little will they know how all the ingredients are natural and wholesome.

Ingredients

60ml (½ cup) Strawberry Chia Jam (see page 56)

dry ingredients

- 150g (1½ cups) ground almonds
- 260g (2 cups) buckwheat flour
- 1 tsp baking powder
- ½ tsp ground ginger
- ½ tsp ground cinnamon
- a pinch of pink Himalayan salt or sea salt

wet ingredients

- 125ml (½ cup) coconut oil, melted
- 125ml (½ cup) maple syrup
- 1 tsp organic vanilla extract
- 1 tsp vanilla powder

1. Preheat the oven to 170°C/325°F/gas 3 and line two large baking sheets with greaseproof paper.
2. In a large mixing bowl, mix together the dry ingredients with a pinch of salt.
3. Combine the wet ingredients and pour into the dry ingredients and mix until a dough forms. If the mixture is a little wet, place in the fridge to chill and firm up.
4. Flour a clean surface and roll the dough out to 5mm thick. Use a 4cm circular cookie cutter or a glass to cut 50 circles out of the dough, re-rolling as needed.
5. Use a small heart-shaped cookie cutter to cut out small hearts in the centre of 25 of the pastry circles, then carefully place all of them on the lined baking sheets (use a spatula or palette knife to do this to stop them breaking).
6. Bake in the hot oven for 10-12 minutes or until lightly golden. Allow to cool before adding ½ teaspoon of jam to the centre of each plain biscuit and topping with the cut-out heart biscuits.

Tip ... If you don't have a cookie cutter, use a knife to cut out little heart shapes.

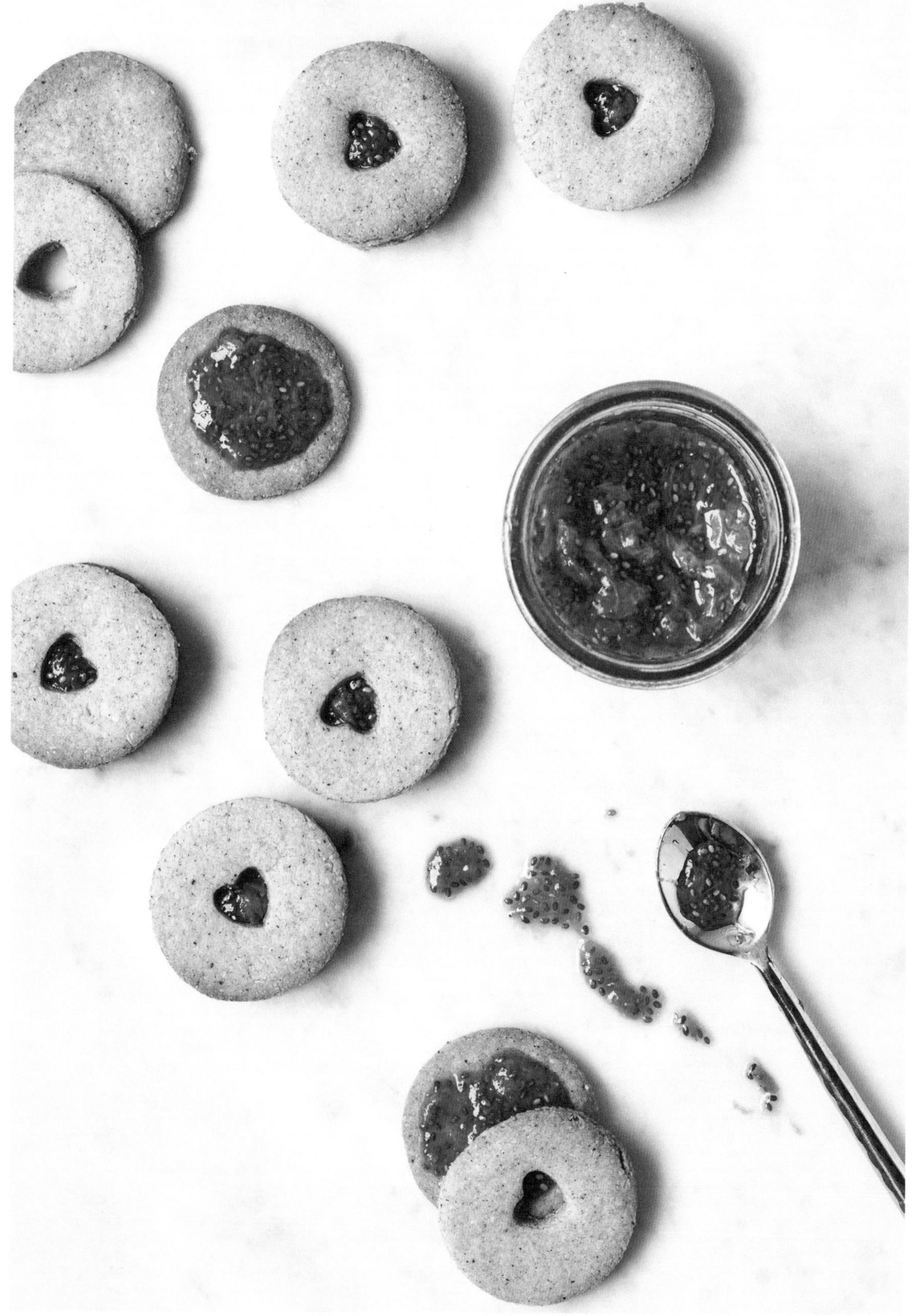

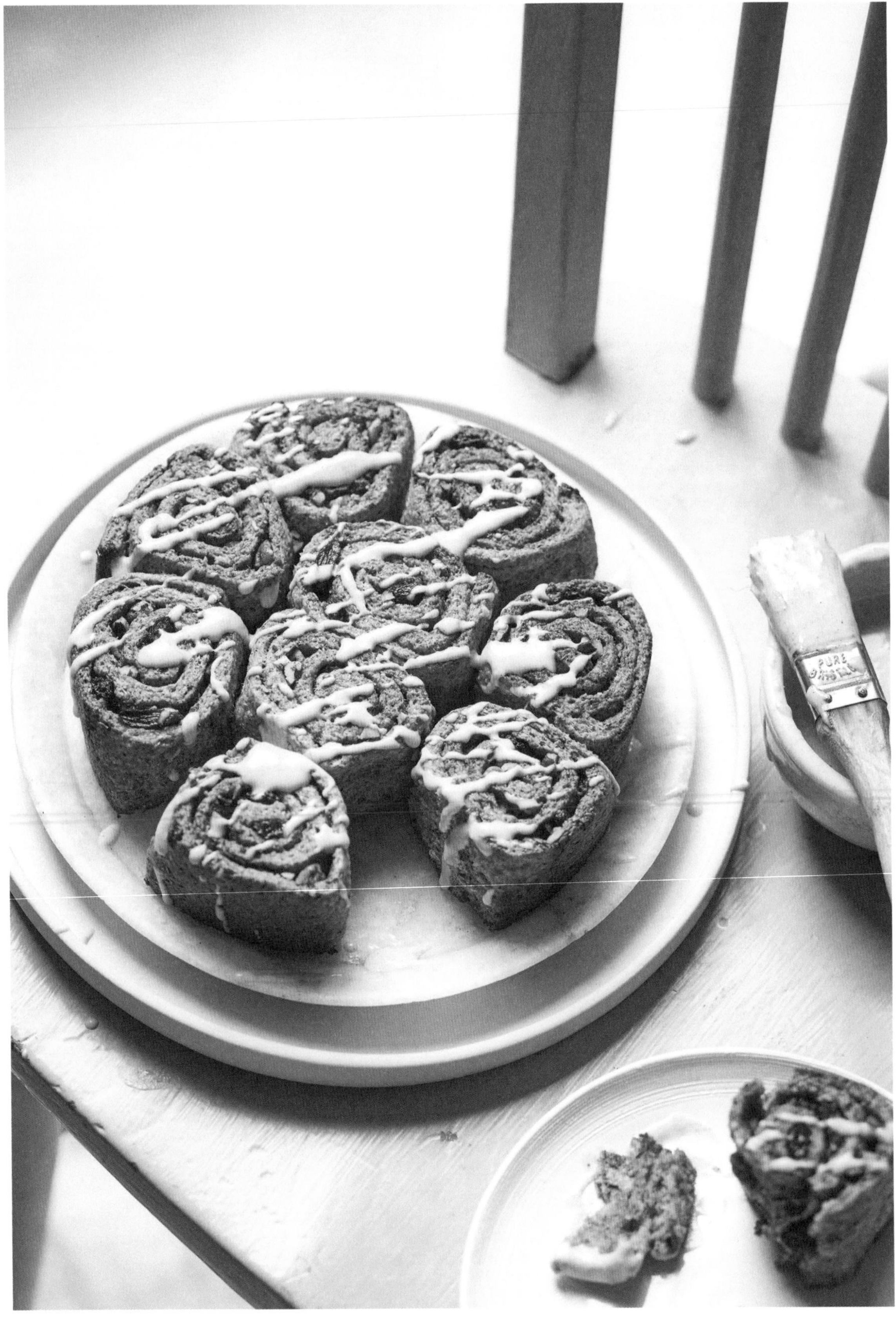
PURE BRISTLE

CINNAMON PECAN ROLLS WITH MAPLE GLAZE

Makes 10

I travel to the US a lot and I always see cinnamon rolls in cafés and bakeries – and I don't blame them! I wanted to create a plant-based version so I could serve these up for the festive season. To avoid the usual large amounts of butter and milk, I've combined it with coconut oil.

Ingredients

dough

- 2 tbsp milled flaxseed
- 250ml (1 cup) unsweetened almond milk
- 285g (1⅞ cups) wholewheat flour
- 150g (1⅓ cups) spelt flour
- 3 tbsp coconut sugar
- 2 tsp quick-action yeast or 1 x 7g sachet
- ½ tsp organic vanilla extract
- 1 tbsp olive oil

filling

- 30ml (⅛ cup) coconut oil
- 40ml (⅙ cup) maple syrup
- 1 tbsp ground cinnamon
- 30g (¼ cup) sultanas
- 50g (½ cup) chopped unsalted raw pecan nuts

1. Mix the flaxseed with 3 tablespoons of water and set aside to thicken. Meanwhile, heat the almond milk in a saucepan over a low heat until slightly warmed but not hot.
2. Mix together the flours, sugar and yeast in a large bowl. Stir the vanilla extract into the warm milk, and create a well in the middle of the dry ingredients. Pour into the well and stir in the flaxseed mixture and the oil.
3. Combine all the ingredients and knead the dough on a lightly floured surface for about 5 minutes. If the dough feels too wet, add an extra tablespoon of spelt flour.
4. Cover the bowl with cling film and keep in a warm place for 1-2 hours or until doubled in size.
5. For the filling, melt the coconut oil in a small saucepan over a low heat. Add the maple syrup, cinnamon, sultanas and pecans and remove from the heat.
6. Flour a clean surface and roll out the dough into a large rectangle shape, about 45cm x 30cm.
7. Spread the filling onto the dough evenly, leaving about 2cm free around the edges.
8. Roll the dough from one long edge to form a log shape. Seal the edge by dipping your finger in water, wetting one side and gently pressing the edges together.

(recipe continues overleaf)

maple glaze
25g (¼ cup) unsalted raw pecan nuts
2 tbsp maple syrup
60ml (¼ cup) unsweetened almond milk
1 tbsp coconut oil
a pinch of pink Himalayan salt or sea salt

9. Use a sharp knife to slice off and discard about 2cm from each end. Slice the rest of the log into 4cm round slices (you should get ten).

10. Place each roll face up in a medium 20cm round baking tin, lightly greased with coconut oil, packed in tightly. Leave to prove for a further 30 minutes or until slightly risen and puffed up.

11. Preheat the oven to 180°C/350°F/gas 4.

12. Bake for 30 minutes, until nicely browned. Remove from the oven and allow to cool while you make the maple glaze.

13. Blend together all the glaze ingredients until totally smooth. Keep in the fridge for a few minutes to set, then drizzle generously over the rolls.

Tip ... I use flaxseed mixed with water to replace eggs in baking recipes. Or I sometimes simply add a tablespoon to my smoothies in the morning for the added health kick.

ONE-DISH BAKED COOKIES

Serves 4

Growing up I used to love going to the supermarket and buying ready-made cookie dough as a treat. We would bring it home, squeeze the dough into a tray and pop it in the oven. This is my take on a guilty pleasure, which can be eaten straight from the tin, yet still using wholesome ingredients.

Ingredients

- 60ml (¼ cup) coconut oil, plus extra, for greasing
- 100g (1 cup) rolled oats
- 100g (1 cup) ground almonds
- 50g (¼ cup) coconut sugar or brown sugar
- 1 tsp baking powder
- 60ml (¼ cup) unsweetened apple sauce
- 60ml (¼ cup) unsweetened almond milk
- 1 tsp organic vanilla extract
- 100g (½ cup) dark chocolate chips
- a pinch of pink Himalayan salt

1. Preheat the oven to 180°C/350°F/gas 4. Grease a 20cm square baking tin with some coconut oil and line with greaseproof paper.
2. Whizz the oats in a food processor to a fine flour and transfer to a large bowl. Mix in the ground almonds, sugar and baking powder with a pinch of salt.
3. Melt the coconut oil in a medium saucepan over a low heat and pour into the bowl of dry ingredients along with the apple sauce, almond milk and vanilla extract, stirring to combine.
4. Stir in the chocolate chips, pour the mixture into the lined baking tin and smooth the top. Bake for 15-20 minutes in the hot oven or until golden. Divide into 4 square cookies or if you can't wait, like me, eat straight from the tin!

BLACK BEAN BANANA BROWNIES

Makes 8

When I first made these I asked my friends to guess the secret ingredient ... they had no idea it was black beans. They have a great consistency, perfect for binding the mixture together. I love that they have a similar richness but are higher in protein and more filling than most traditional brownies, so they are perfect for a post-gym treat.

Ingredients

- coconut oil, for greasing
- 2 ripe bananas, peeled
- 1 x 400g tin black beans, drained
- 30g (¼ cup) raw cacao powder
- 30g (¼ cup) brown rice flour
- 60g (¼ cup) almond butter
- 125ml (½ cup) agave nectar or maple syrup
- 60ml (½ cup) unsweetened almond milk
- ½ tsp baking powder
- 1 tsp organic vanilla extract
- 25g (¼ cup) unsalted raw walnuts, plus 5 to top

1. Preheat the oven to 180°C/350°F/gas 4. Grease a 21cm x 10cm baking tray with coconut oil and line with greaseproof paper.

2. Add all the ingredients apart from the walnuts to a food processor and blend until smooth.

3. Add the walnuts to the mixture and blend for a couple of seconds until the walnuts have broken down into chunks (or use bought chopped walnuts and stir in).

4. Pour the mixture into the tray, then crush the remaining 5 walnuts and sprinkle over the brownie mixture. Bake in the hot oven for 20 minutes. Allow to cool fully in the tin before slicing into eight squares.

CHOCOLATE CUPCAKES WITH COCONUT CREAM FROSTING

Makes 12

I love cupcakes, but then again who doesn't? I didn't think it would be possible to make a plant-based version that tasted so good, but after many sessions in the kitchen I finally found a mixture of ingredients that worked. The rich coconut cream frosting is so delicious and very tempting to eat straight from the bowl.

Ingredients

260g (1½ cups) brown rice flour
60g (½ cup) raw cacao powder
½ tsp bicarbonate of soda
1 tsp baking powder
250g (1 cup) plain coconut yoghurt
100g (½ cup) coconut sugar
180ml (¾ cup) unsweetened almond milk
1 tsp organic vanilla extract
1 tsp apple cider vinegar

coconut cream frosting

½ x 400g tin coconut milk, refrigerated
2 tbsp raw cacao powder, plus extra for dusting
2 tbsp maple syrup
½ tsp organic vanilla extract
½ tsp arrowroot powder
2 tbsp raw cacao nibs, to decorate

1. Preheat the oven to 180°C/350°F/gas 4 and line one or two muffin tins with 12 paper cupcake cases.
2. Start by mixing the rice flour, cacao powder, bicarbonate of soda and baking powder together in a bowl and set aside.
3. In a separate large bowl, use an electric hand whisk to whip the coconut yoghurt together with the coconut sugar and gradually add the almond milk, whisking as you pour. Fold in the vanilla extract and apple cider vinegar.
4. Gradually fold the dry ingredients into the wet ingredients, making sure they are fully combined but avoiding mixing too much.
5. Divide the mixture between the cupcake cases and bake in the hot oven for 25 minutes, or until cooked through. To check whether the cakes are cooked, insert a knife into the centre of one cake – if the knife comes out clean they are done; if still sticky, return to the oven and bake for a further 5 minutes or until a knife inserted comes out clean. Remove from the oven and allow the cakes to cool on a wire rack.

(recipe continues overleaf)

6. While the cupcakes are cooling, make the coconut cream frosting. Scoop out the solid coconut cream that has risen to the top of the tin of coconut milk (this should be around 150g) and place in a large bowl. Use an electric hand whisk to whisk all the ingredients together until thickened and the bowl can be turned upside down without the mixture moving. If it's not thick enough, keep in the fridge for about 20 minutes before spreading on the cupcakes.

7. Once the cupcakes have totally cooled (this is important), smoothly spread the coconut cream frosting onto each cake. Finish with a dusting of cacao powder and a sprinkling of cacao nibs over the cakes. Keep refrigerated in an airtight container.

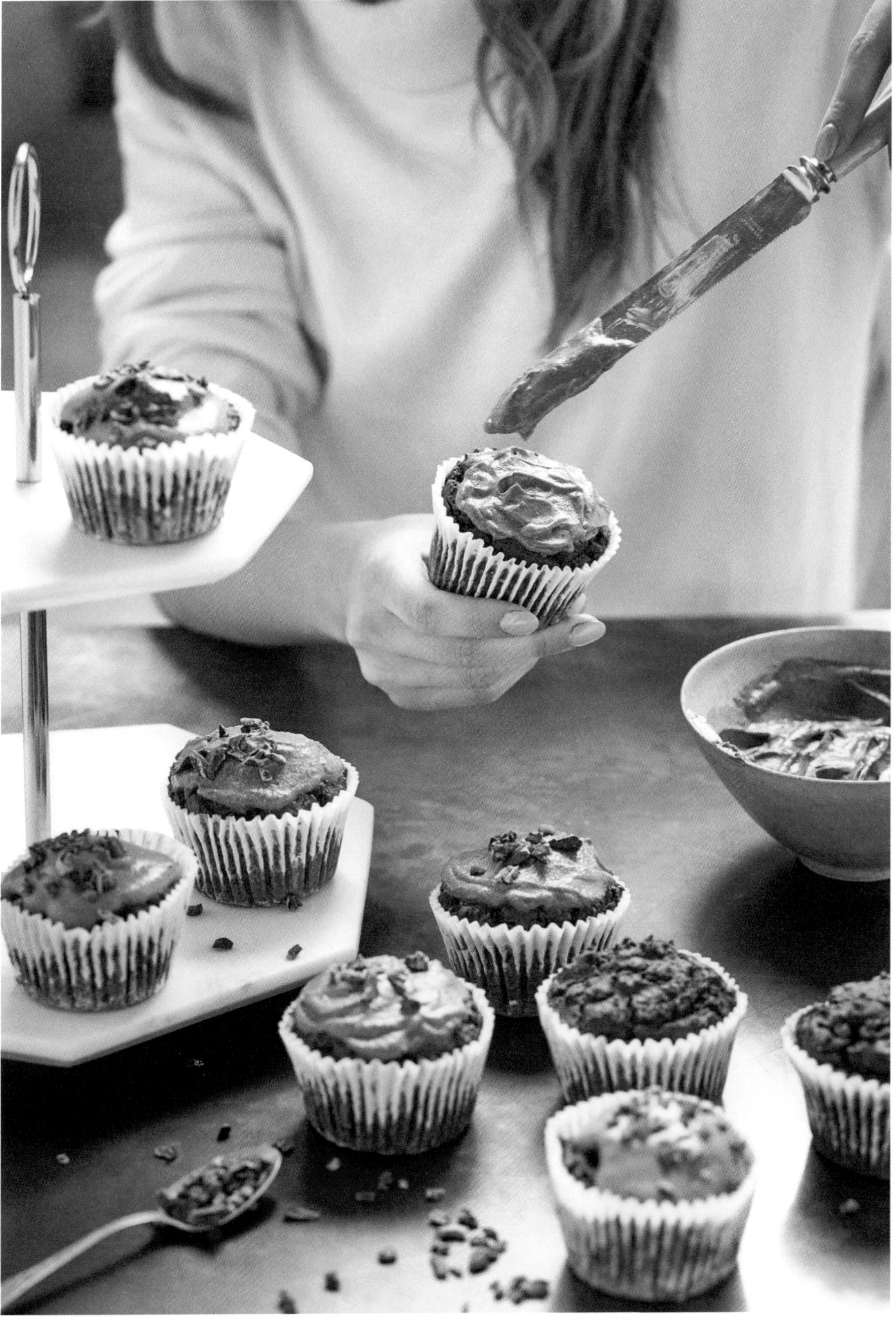

DATE, WALNUT + BANANA LOAF

Serves 10

One of my favourite things to do with friends is share afternoon tea; it's a great way to see old friends and gossip over cake. This loaf is perfect for slicing up and sharing. There's something very wholesome about the combination of banana and date, with the added crunch from the walnuts.

Ingredients

- **coconut oil, for greasing**
- **2½ ripe bananas, peeled**
- **200g (1½ cups) buckwheat flour**
- **25g (¼ cup) chopped unsalted raw walnuts**
- **1 tsp baking powder**
- **1 tsp bicarbonate of soda**
- **110g (⅔ cup) deglet nour dates, pitted and chopped**
- **190ml (¾ cup) unsweetened almond milk**
- **a pinch of Himalayan pink salt or sea salt**

1. Preheat the oven to 170°C/325°F/gas 3 and grease an 18cm x 8cm loaf tin with a little coconut oil and line with greaseproof paper.
2. Mash 2 bananas and slice the remaining half-banana.
3. In a large bowl, combine the flour, walnuts, baking powder, bicarbonate of soda and a pinch of salt.
4. Stir in the mashed and sliced bananas and chopped dates and slowly add the almond milk until the mixture is fully combined.
5. Pour the mixture into the tin and bake in the hot oven for 35-40 minutes or until golden and cooked through. To check whether the loaf is cooked, insert a knife into the centre of the loaf – if it comes out clean it is done, if still sticky, return to the oven and bake for a further 15 minutes or until a knife inserted comes out clean.
6. Allow to cool in the tin for 10 minutes before turning out onto a wire rack to cool completely.

Serving ideas...

Try spreading a slice with almond butter or one of my homemade chia jams (see page 56).

CARROT CAKE LOAF + LEMON 'CREAM CHEESE'

Serves 10

Baking has always been part of my upbringing. It has this wonderful way of getting the whole family into the kitchen, and carrot cake is one of my favourites. Just remember, cake doesn't have to be bad for you, it's about what you throw into the mixing bowl!

Ingredients

- 120ml (½ cup) melted coconut oil, plus extra for greasing
- 130g (1 cup) spelt flour
- 115g (1 cup) almond flour
- 90g (¾ cup) unsalted raw walnuts, chopped
- 60g (½ cup) raisins
- 1 tsp ground cinnamon
- ½ tsp ground nutmeg
- ½ tsp ground ginger
- 2 tsp baking powder
- 1 tsp bicarbonate of soda
- 2 small carrots, peeled and finely grated (you need 115g)
- 120ml (½ cup) unsweetened almond milk
- 120ml (½ cup) maple syrup
- 1 tsp vanilla powder or 2 teaspoons organic vanilla extract
- 1 tsp apple cider vinegar

topping

- 80g (½ cup) unsalted raw cashew nuts, soaked
- 1 tbsp coconut nectar or maple syrup
- ½ tsp vanilla powder
- 3-5 tbsp unsweetened almond milk
- ½ lemon

1. Preheat the oven to 180°C/350°F/gas 4. Grease a 18.5cm x 8.5cm loaf tin with coconut oil and line with greaseproof paper.

2. In a large mixing bowl, combine the flours, 80g walnuts, raisins, spices, baking powder, bicarbonate of soda and 100g grated carrot. Toss well to combine thoroughly. This is key, or all your fruit and nuts will sink to the bottom of the loaf! In another bowl combine the almond milk, coconut oil, maple syrup, vanilla and vinegar (this helps with the rise).

3. Add the wet ingredients to the dry and mix until fully combined. Spoon into the lined tin and bake in the hot oven for 60-70 minutes, until cooked through and nicely browned on top. (Don't be tempted to open the oven door before the baking time is done.) Remove from the oven, leave to cool in the tin for 20 minutes, then place on a cooling rack and leave to cool completely.

4. Drain the cashews and place in a food processor. Pulse until the nuts are broken up. Add the coconut nectar, vanilla powder and almond milk. Finely grate in the lemon zest and add a squeeze of juice. Blend for a few minutes until smooth and creamy, adding more milk if necessary.

5. Transfer into a bowl and refrigerate for 10 minutes, while the cake cools.

6. Spoon the topping onto the cooled cake and sprinkle the remaining chopped walnuts and grated carrots on top.

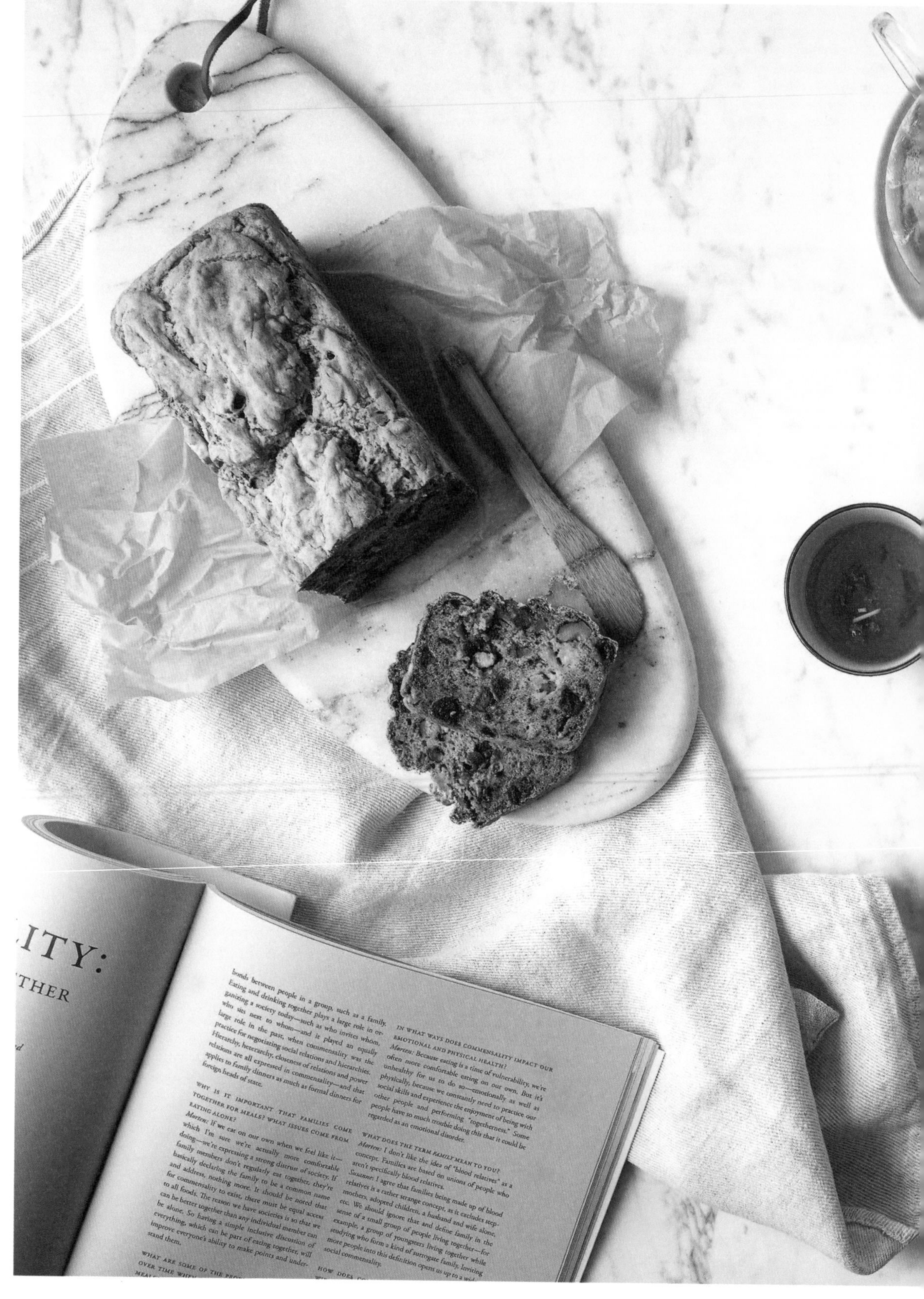
ITY:
THER
bonds between people in a group, such as a family. Eating and drinking together plays a large role in organizing a society today—such as who invites whom, who sits next to whom—and it played an equally large role in the past, when commensality was the practice for negotiating social relations and hierarchies. Hierarchy, heterarchy, closeness of relations and power relations are all expressed in commensality—and that applies to family dinners as much as formal dinners for foreign heads of state.
WHY IS IT IMPORTANT THAT FAMILIES COME TOGETHER FOR MEALS? WHAT ISSUES COME FROM EATING ALONE?
Morten: If we eat on our own when we feel like it—which I'm sure we're actually more comfortable doing—we're expressing a strong distrust of society. If family members don't regularly eat together, they're basically declaring the family to be a common name and address, nothing more. It should be noted that for commensality to exist, there must be equal access to all foods. The reason we have societies is so that we can be better together than any individual member can be alone. So having a simple inclusive discussion of everything, which can be part of eating together, will improve everyone's ability to make points and understand them.
IN WHAT WAYS DOES COMMENSALITY IMPACT OUR EMOTIONAL AND PHYSICAL HEALTH?
Morten: Because eating is a time of vulnerability, we're often more comfortable eating on our own. But it's unhealthy for us to do so—emotionally as well as physically, because we constantly need to practice our social skills and experience the enjoyment of being with other people and performing "togetherness." Some people have so much trouble doing this that it could be regarded as an emotional disorder.
WHAT DOES THE TERM FAMILY MEAN TO YOU?
Morten: I don't like the idea of "blood relatives" as a concept. Families are based on unions of people who aren't specifically blood relatives.
Susanne: I agree that families being made up of blood relatives is a rather strange concept, as it excludes stepmothers, adopted children, a husband and wife alone, etc. We should ignore that and define family in the sense of a small group of people living together—for example, a group of youngsters living together while studying who form a kind of surrogate family. Inviting more people into this definition opens us up to a wider social commensality.

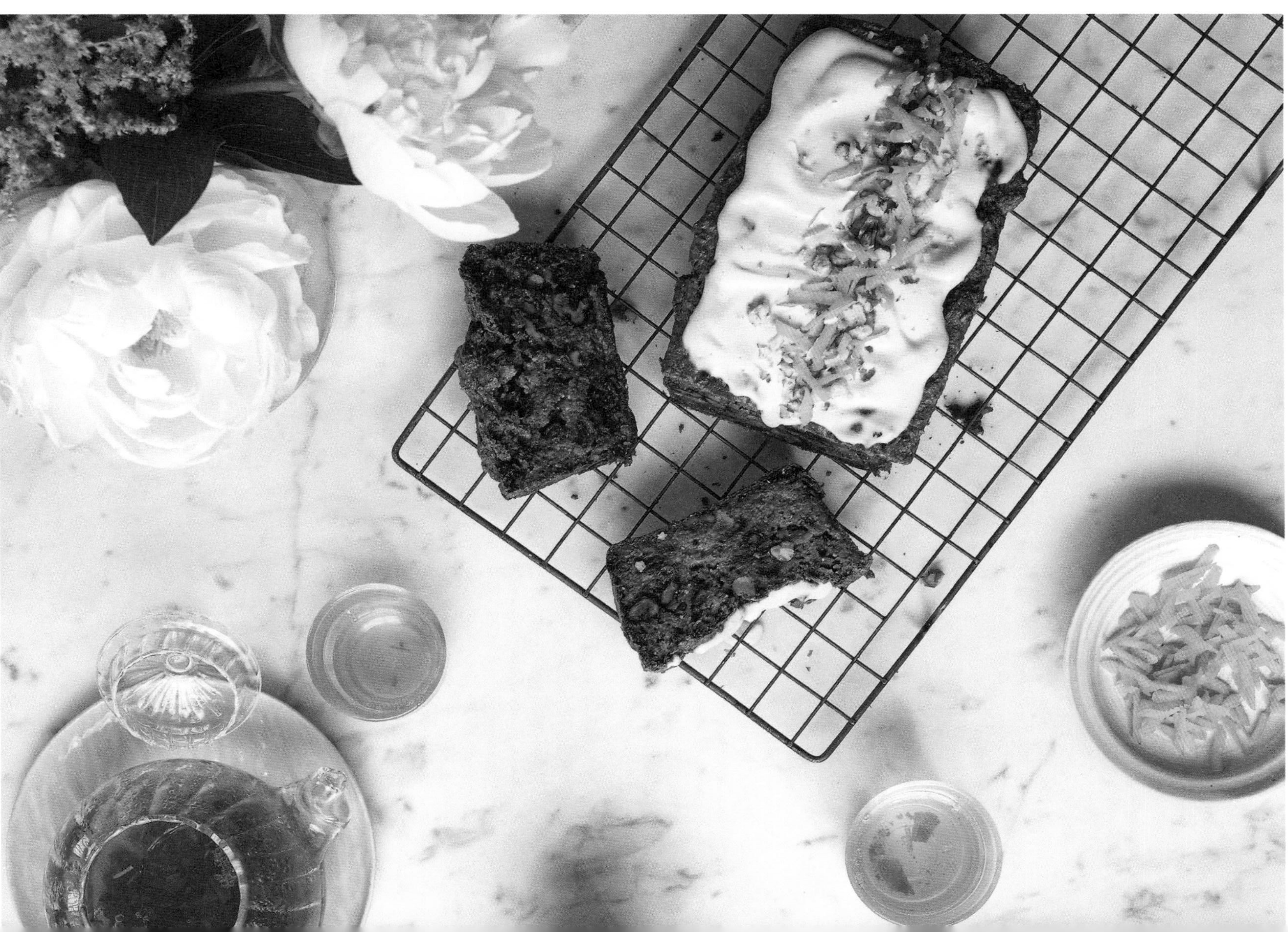

BEETROOT CAKE WITH CHOCOLATE GANACHE

Serves 10

Don't knock this until you try it. Even if you don't like beetroot, you won't be able to taste the earthiness once it's mixed with chocolate – and the ganache means your friends won't guess it's plant-based. If you want to make a birthday cake for a friend, this will seriously impress.

Ingredients

wet ingredients

- 125ml (½ cup) coconut oil, plus extra for greasing
- 300g (1½ cups) apple sauce
- 500ml (2 cups) unsweetened almond milk
- 1 tsp apple cider vinegar

dry ingredients

- 100g (1 cup) rolled oats
- 400g (2¼ cups) brown rice flour
- 150g (1½) cups coconut sugar
- 80g (⅔ cup) raw cacao powder
- 2 tsp baking powder
- 1 tsp bicarbonate of soda
- 3 medium beetroot, peeled and finely grated
- a pinch of pink Himalayan salt or sea salt

chocolate ganache

- 100g dark chocolate, 70% cocoa solids (dairy-free)
- 155g (1 cup) unsalted raw cashews, soaked overnight
- 185ml (¾ cup) unsweetened almond milk

1. Preheat the oven to 180°C/350°F/gas 4. Grease two 20cm sandwich cake tins with coconut oil.
2. Melt the coconut oil in a small saucepan over a low heat.
3. Grind the oats to a flour in a food processor, tip into a large bowl and mix with the rest of the dry ingredients, except the beetroot. In a separate bowl, mix together the melted coconut oil with the remaining wet ingredients.
4. Make a well in the middle of the dry ingredients and fold in the wet mixture until fully combined. Stir in the grated beetroot, keeping aside 2 tablespoons for later.
5. Divide the mixture evenly between the cake tins and bake for 30 minutes or until a knife inserted comes out clean. Carefully tip out onto a cooling rack and allow to cool.
6. To make the chocolate ganache, break up the dark chocolate and place in a heatproof bowl. Set this above a saucepan of water simmering over a low heat to melt.
7. Drain the cashews and blend with the almond milk until smooth, then tip into a bowl.
8. Stir the melted chocolate into the cashew and almond milk and place in the fridge to firm up for 20 minutes.
9. Spread a third of the ganache onto one of the cooled cakes. Place the other cake on top and smooth the remaining ganache over the top and sides with a palette knife.
10. Decorate with the reserved grated beetroot and a dusting of cacao or a grating of chocolate, if you like.

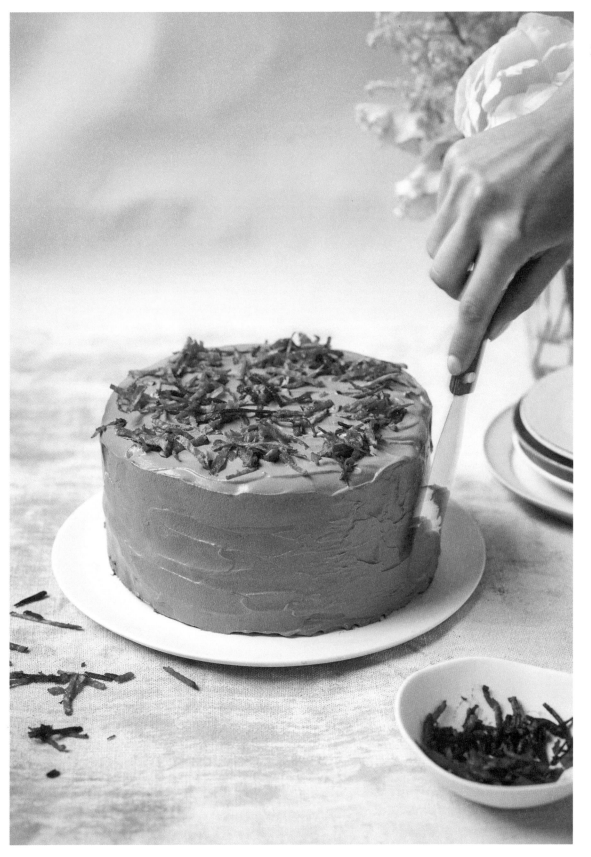

FLAPJACKS – 3 WAYS

Flapjacks are a delicious coffee-shop staple but are almost always made with sugar, syrup and artificial sweeteners. I love the taste, though, so I had to make my own healthy version. I make a batch if I'm having my girlfriends over, and they are even great as a grab-and-go breakfast.

BLUEBERRY + COCONUT

Makes 12

Ingredients

3 ripe bananas, peeled
300g (3 cups) rolled oats
90g (1 cup) desiccated coconut
150g (1 cup) blueberries
90ml (⅓ cup) coconut oil, plus extra for greasing
50g (¼ cup) coconut sugar

1. Preheat the oven to 180°C/350°F/ gas 4. Lightly grease a deep 20cm square baking tin with coconut oil and line with greaseproof paper.
2. Mash the bananas with the back of a fork until smooth and set aside.
3. Mix together the oats and desiccated coconut in a large bowl and stir in the blueberries.
4. Melt the coconut oil in a small saucepan over a low heat. Add the coconut sugar and stir for a couple of minutes to dissolve, then stir in the mashed bananas.
5. Add to the bowl of dry ingredients and stir to totally combine.
6. Pour into the tin, smooth the top with the back of a wooden spoon and bake in the hot oven for 30 minutes, until golden.
7. While still warm, slice into 12 squares and allow to cool in the tin. Once cooled, keep in an airtight container. Perfect for a grab-and-go snack!

BANANA, SULTANA + THYME

Makes 12

Ingredients

90ml (⅓ cup) coconut oil, plus extra for greasing
3 ripe bananas, peeled
150g (1 cup) unsalted raw almonds
300g (3 cups) rolled oats
60g (½ cup) sultanas
12 fresh thyme sprigs, leaves picked or 2 tsp dried thyme
3 tbsp coconut sugar

1. Preheat the oven to 180°C/350°F/gas 4. Lightly grease a deep 20cm square baking tin with coconut oil and line with greaseproof paper.
2. Mash 2 of the bananas with the back of a fork and slice the other one.
3. Crush the almonds in a pestle and mortar into small chunks and mix with the oats and sultanas in a large bowl.
4. Roughly chop the thyme sprigs and stir about 2 tablespoons of the leaves into the oats.
5. Melt the coconut oil in a small saucepan over a low heat. Remove from the heat, stir in the mashed bananas and coconut sugar, then mix into the oats with the sliced banana.
6. Pour the mixture into the tin. Use the back of a wooden spoon to press the mixture down and bake for 25 minutes in the hot oven until golden.
7. While still warm, slice into squares and allow to cool in the tin. Once cooled, keep in an airtight container.

PEANUT BUTTER + JAM

Makes 12

Ingredients

coconut oil, for greasing
2 ripe bananas, peeled
250g (1 cup) crunchy peanut butter
125ml (½ cup) unsweetened almond milk
40g (¼ cup) coconut sugar
300g (3 cups) rolled oats
250ml (1 cup) Strawberry Chia Jam (see page 56), or 100% fruit strawberry jam, refrigerated

1. Preheat the oven to 180°C/350°F/gas 4. Lightly grease a medium 20cm square baking tin with a little coconut oil and line with greaseproof paper.
2. Mash the bananas with a fork until smooth and place in a large mixing bowl. Stir in the peanut butter, almond milk and coconut sugar. Once all the ingredients are combined, stir in the oats.
3. Pour a little more than half of the mixture into the tin. Use the back of a spoon to compress the mixture down evenly and bake in the hot oven for 15 minutes.
4. Pour over the jam and smooth down. Now add the remaining flapjack mixture by adding about a tablespoon at a time over the top. This layer is just rough, so don't worry about trying to smooth it down. You will be able to see patches of jam.
5. Bake in the hot oven for a further 20-25 minutes until golden.
6. Remove from the oven and while still warm, cut into 12, but allow to cool for about 10 minutes before removing from the tray.

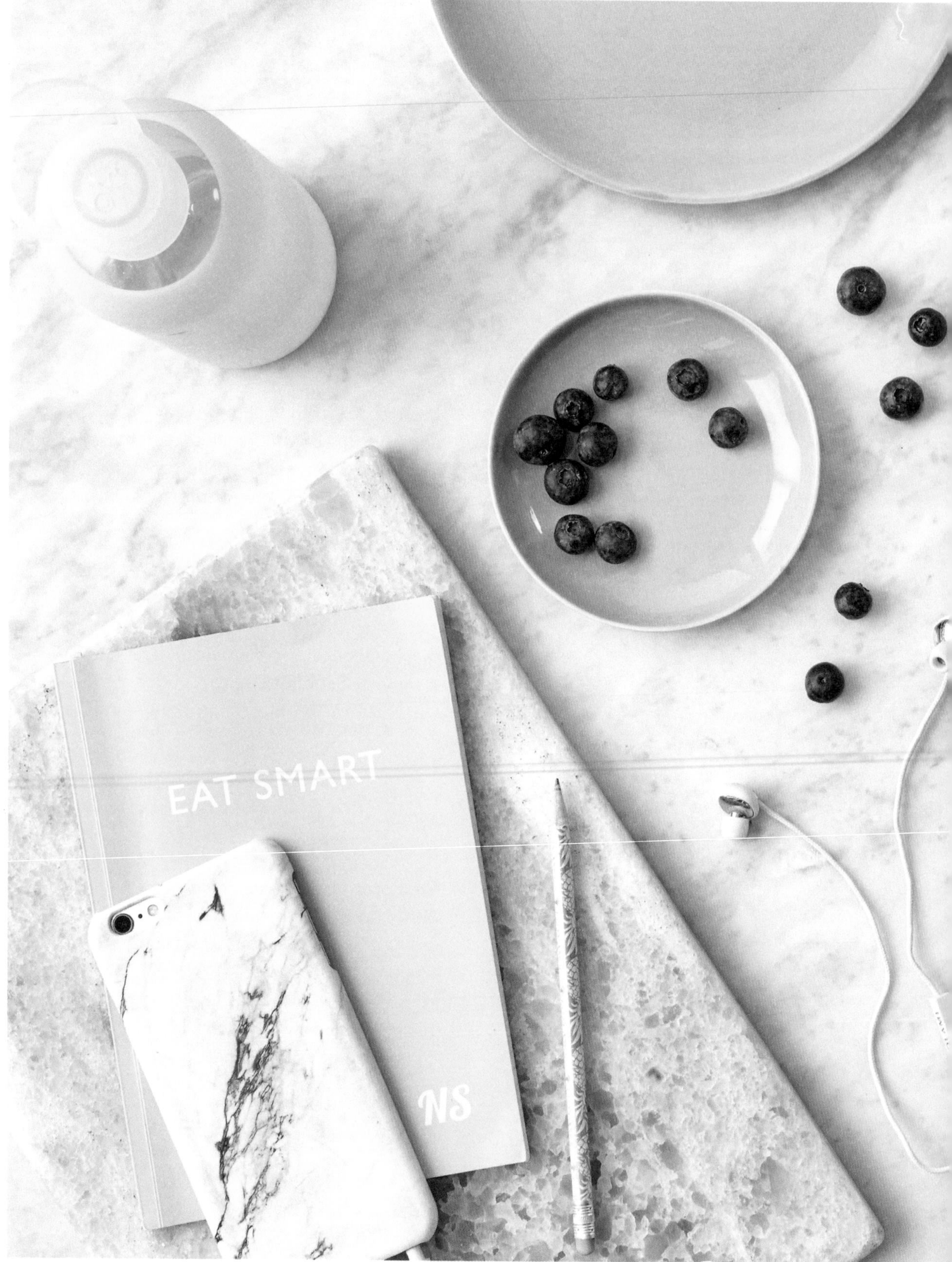
EAT SMART
NS

Drinks

06

HOMEMADE REFRESHING LEMONADE

Makes 1 litre

When my mum had a baby shower for my little sister I wanted to provide a delicious non-alcoholic drink. As it was the height of summer I decided on a refreshing homemade lemonade to cool everyone down, sweetened with natural agave nectar or honey.

Ingredients

2.5cm piece of fresh ginger, peeled and sliced
4 tbsp runny honey or agave nectar
¼ bunch of fresh mint, leaves picked
6 lemons

1. Bring 1 litre (4 cups) of water to the boil in a large saucepan, then turn down to a low heat.
2. Add the ginger to the water with the honey or agave nectar, 5 mint leaves and the juice from 5 of the lemons (about 200ml/¾ cup juice). Leave for 20 minutes on a very low heat for the flavours to infuse.
3. Strain the lemonade into a jug, discard the ginger and mint and keep the lemonade to one side to cool. Chill in the fridge for at least 1–2 hours or until cold.
4. Slice the remaining lemon and serve the chilled lemonade with ice cubes, lemon slices and the remaining fresh mint leaves.

Tip ... To get the most juice from the lemons, roll them on a surface before you slice them; this releases the juices.

MOCKTAILS – 3 WAYS

These drinks are perfect for quenching your thirst and cooling you down on a hot summer's day, especially when served ice cold. The Pina Coolada will transport you to a beach in Hawaii, the Virgin Mary to a cocktail bar in New York, and the Cucumber and Melon muddler is fit for a spa.

PINA COOLADA

Serves 1

Ingredients

1 tbsp tinned coconut milk, refrigerated
100g (½ cup) fresh pineapple chunks
250ml (1 cup) coconut water
½ tsp vanilla essence or extract
juice of ½ lime

1. Scoop out 1 tablespoon of the solid coconut cream that has risen to the top of the tin of coconut milk and place in a blender or NutriBullet.
2. Add the remaining ingredients, whizz in the blender and serve in a glass over crushed ice.

CUCUMBER + MELON MUDDLER

Serves 1

Ingredients

½ cucumber, chopped
2 celery sticks
¼ galia melon, deseeded, flesh scooped out and chopped
8 fresh mint leaves, plus 1 sprig to serve
juice of ½ lemon

1. Feed the cucumber, celery, melon and mint through an extractor juicer and pour into a glass with 3 tablespoons water.
2. Squeeze the lemon juice into the glass, stir and serve with the fresh mint sprig.

VIRGIN MARY

Serves 1

Ingredients

4 large ripe vine tomatoes
2 celery sticks, trimmed
juice of ½ lemon
a small pinch of cayenne pepper
pink Himalayan salt or sea salt and freshly ground black pepper

1. Feed the tomatoes and 1 celery stick through an extractor juicer.
2. Stir in the lemon juice and cayenne and serve in a glass with a small celery stick and a pinch of salt and black pepper.

Tip ... To make these into fun cocktails, add 25ml of rum to the Pina Coolada, 25ml of vodka to the Virgin Mary and 25ml of gin to the Cucumber + Melon Muddler.

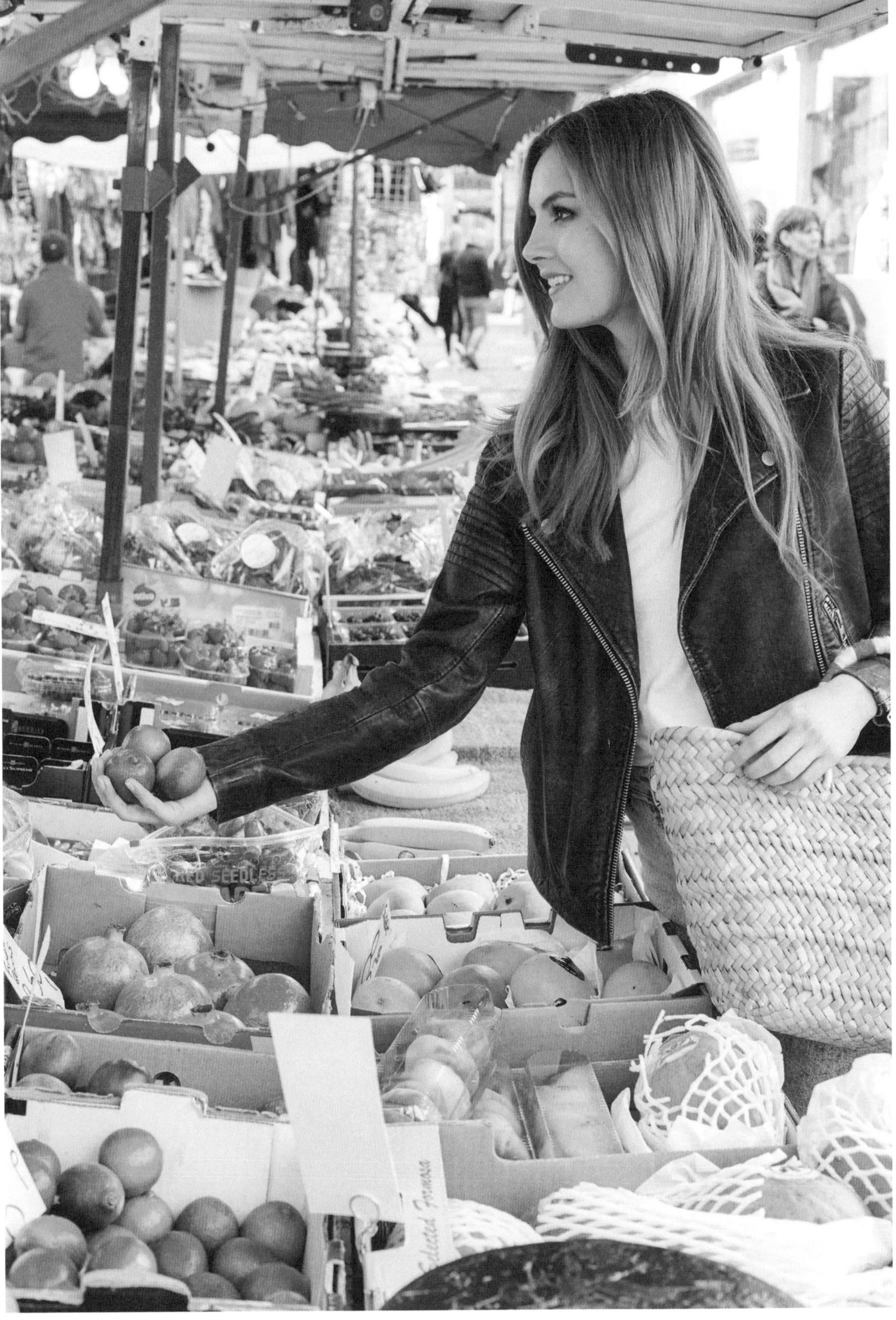
Selected Formosa

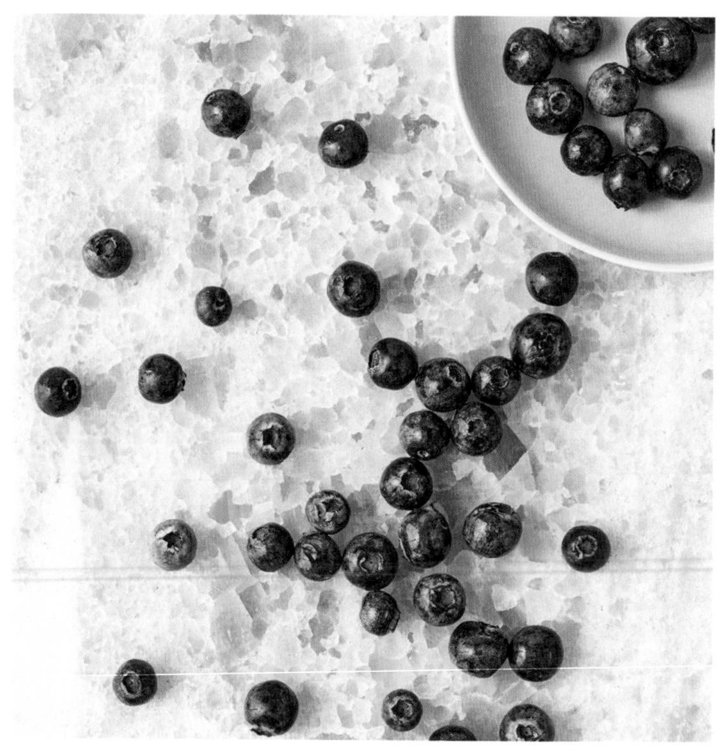

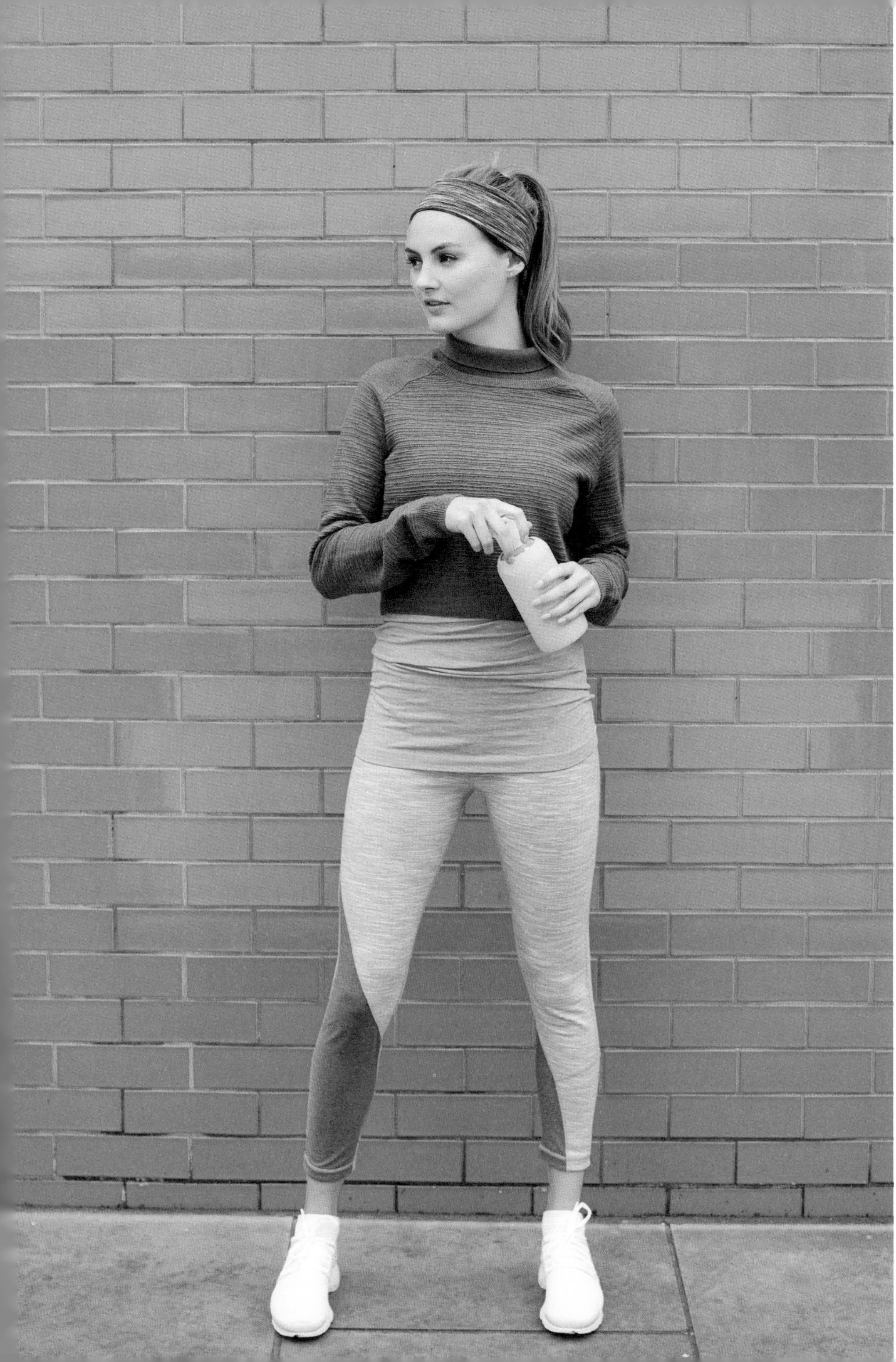

MAPLE MATCHA LATTE

Serves 1

This is a real energy-booster, perfect for an early morning pick-me-up and a great alternative to coffee.

Ingredients

250ml (1 cup) unsweetened almond milk
1 tsp matcha powder
1 tsp maple syrup, plus extra to sweeten
¼ tsp vanilla powder or ½ tsp organic vanilla extract

1. Heat the almond milk in a saucepan over a medium heat until simmering.
2. Add the matcha powder to a mug, pour over 60ml (¼ cup) boiling water, whisk to dissolve and stir in the maple syrup and vanilla powder.
3. Pour the hot milk into a latte glass and stir in the matcha mixture. If using frothed milk, pour the matcha mixture carefully into one side of the glass to keep the milk lovely and frothy, adding extra maple syrup to sweeten, if needed.

Tip ... If you have a milk frothing machine, use this instead get the milk lovely and frothy.

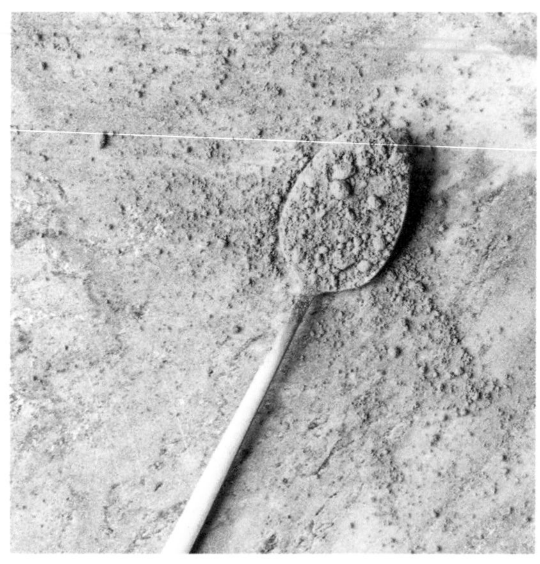

MORNING DETOX WATER

Serves 1

I like to kick-start my days with a hot detox water – the zingy lemon and hot cayenne pepper give a real wake-up kick.

Ingredients

1cm piece of fresh ginger, peeled and sliced
½ tsp ground cinnamon
a pinch of cayenne pepper
1 tsp honey or maple syrup
juice of ½ lemon

1. Add the ginger to a glass with the cinnamon, cayenne pepper and honey. Squeeze in the lemon juice and mix.
2. Top up with boiling water, stir and leave to brew for 5 minutes.

SLEEPY BREW

Serves 1

In the evenings I want a milky drink that calms the body and mind but that's made from incredible ingredients. My recipe uses maca for a slight caramel taste.

Ingredients

250ml (1 cup) unsweetened almond milk
2 teaspoons maca powder
1 tsp barley malt extract
½ tsp vanilla powder or 1 tsp organic vanilla extract

1. Heat the almond milk in a saucepan over a medium heat.
2. Place the maca powder, barley malt extract and vanilla powder in your favourite mug, pour the milk on top, whisk until dissolved and serve.

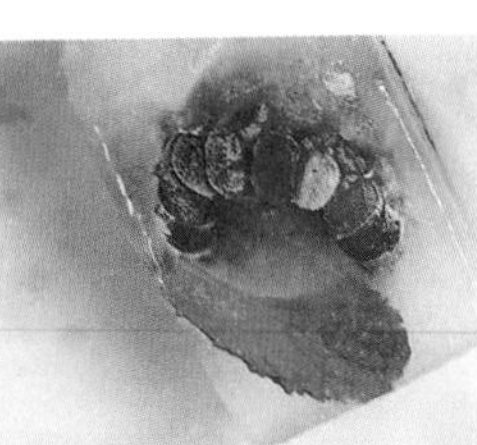

JEWELLED ICE CUBES

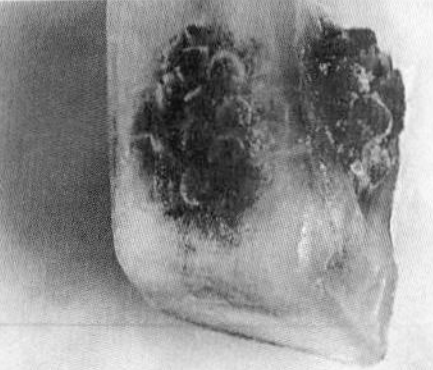

Makes 16 ice cubes (4 of each flavour)

I'm the kind of person who has to really remind myself to drink water throughout the day to keep hydrated. Adding these fruity ice cubes to a glass of water gives it a subtle flavour and looks so beautiful – far more appealing than a glass of plain water.

Ingredients

lime + passion fruit
½ lime, cut into small chunks
1 passion fruit, pulp and seeds scooped out

raspberries + mint
4 raspberries
4 small fresh mint leaves

lemon + blueberry
½ lemon,cut into small chunks
4 blueberries

cucumber + lemon
2cm piece of cucumber, cut into small chunks
½ lemon,cut into small chunks

1. Lay out all the ingredients. Divide among sections of a large ice-cube tray in their combinations to make four of each variety.
2. Top up with water and freeze overnight.
3. These go well served with sparkling water or even with my Homemade Refreshing Lemonade (see page 225).

Tip ... To get crystal-clear ice, boil the water first and allow to cool slightly before pouring into the ice-cube tray.

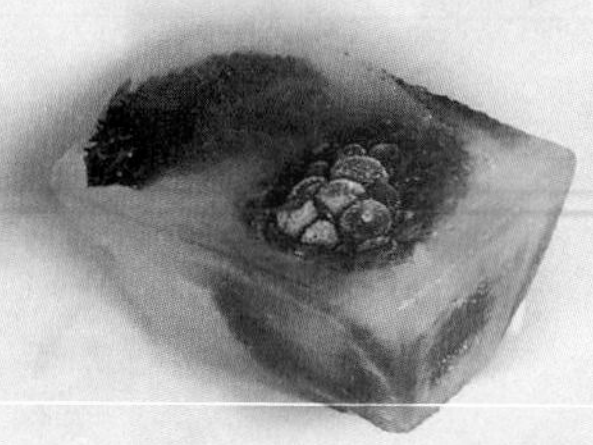

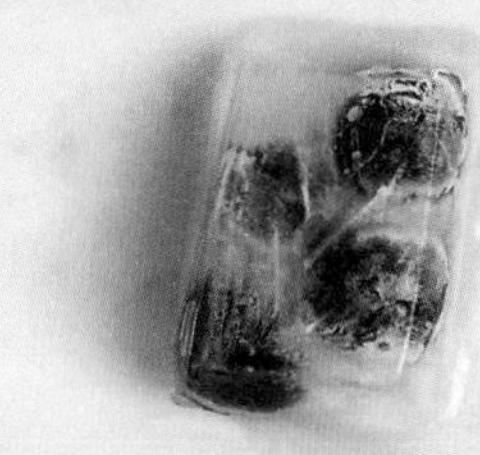

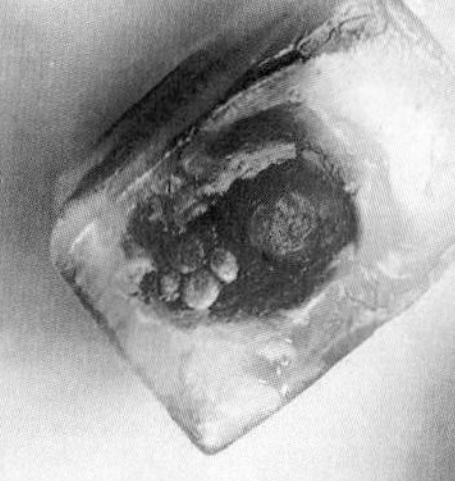

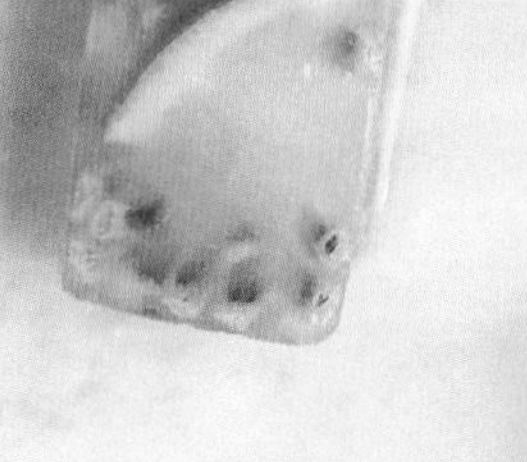

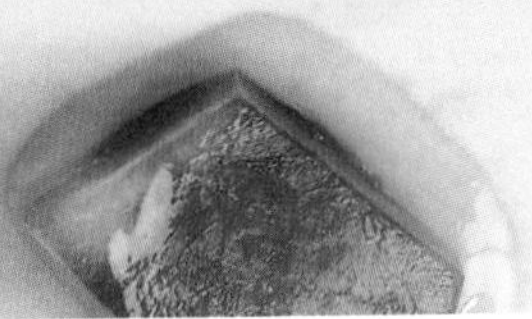

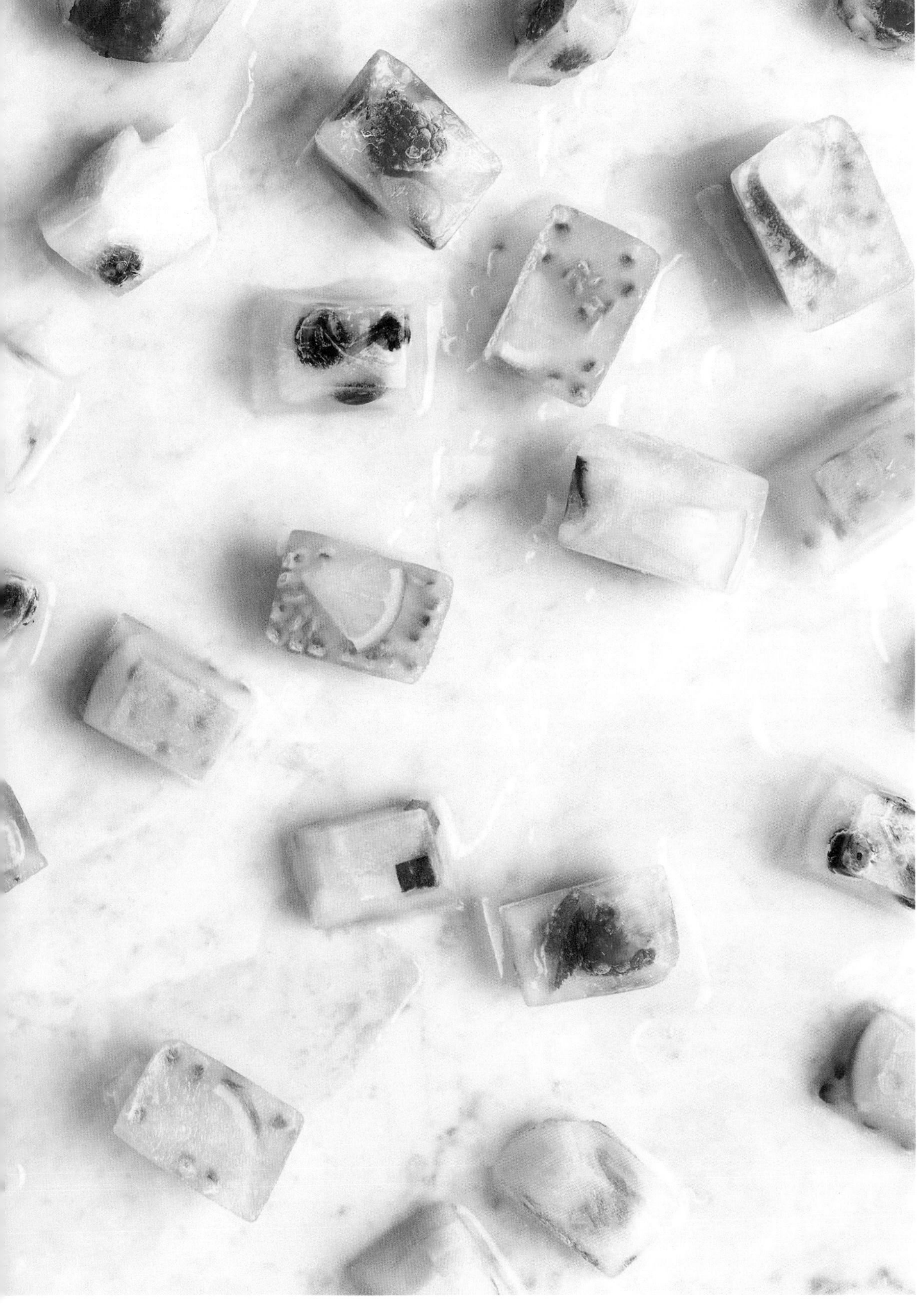

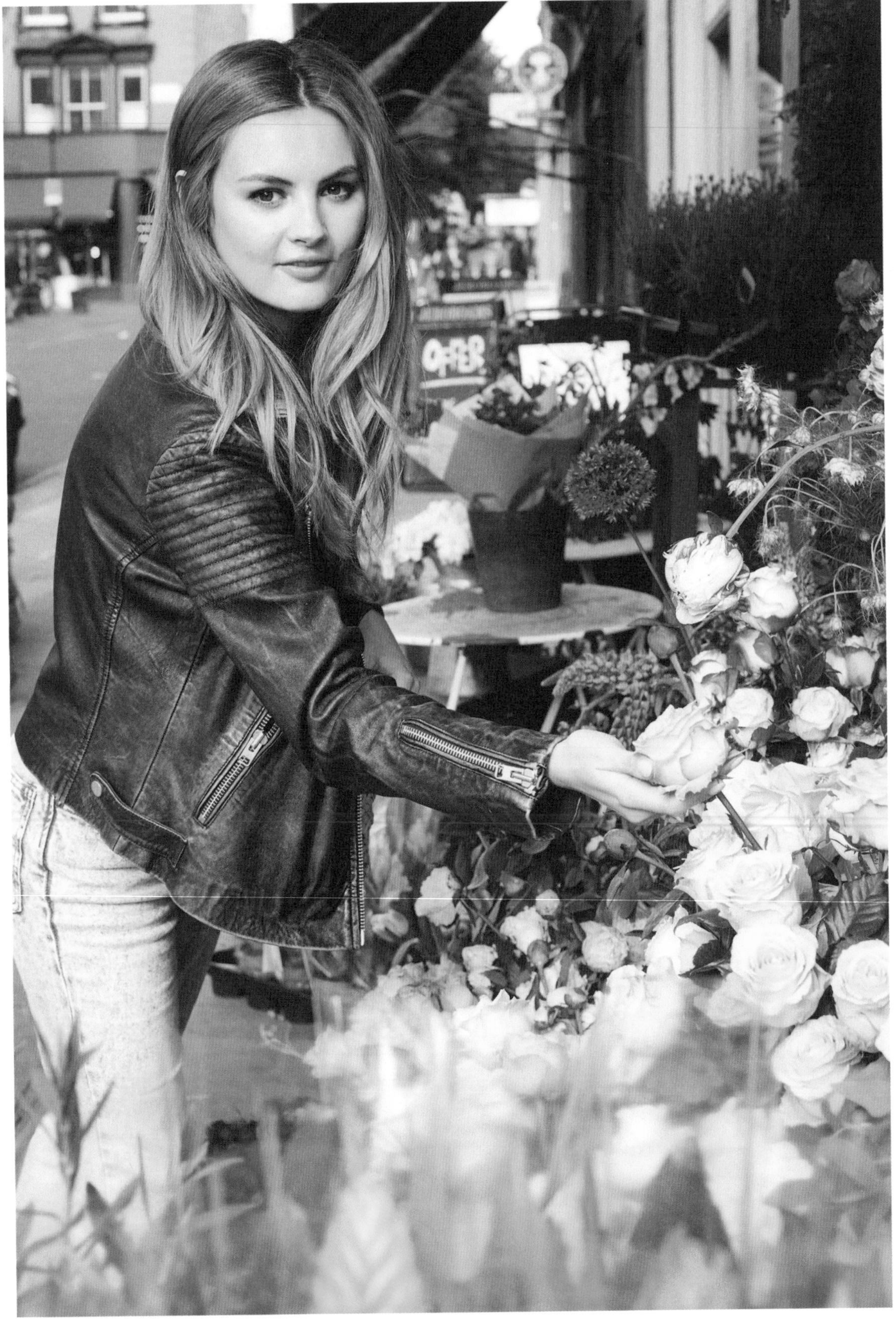
OFFER

SMOOTHIES

If I feel like a lighter breakfast, I opt for a smoothie. They're super quick to make and packed full of nutrients. The Blueberry Swirl and Blackberry Crumble (see page 236) are quite filling, while the Ultimate Carrot, below, and the Mango Passion (see page 236) are refreshing and nourishing. Don't be wary of the beetroot – when blended with berries it tastes incredible.

THE ULTIMATE CARROT SMOOTHIE

Serves 2

Ingredients

carrot

1 large carrot, peeled and chopped
1 large orange, peeled, pith removed and chopped
125ml (½ cup) coconut water
1 tbsp lemon juice

green

½ avocado, peeled and stoned
½ ripe banana, peeled and frozen
a small handful of spinach
60ml (¼ cup) unsweetened almond milk

1. Whizz all the carrot juice ingredients together in a blender and three-quarter fill your glasses. Leave to one side for a couple of minutes for the ingredients to separate – the pulp will naturally rise to the top and this will make it easier for the green smoothie to stay on top.
2. Rinse the blender, then whizz the green juice ingredients together. It will be thick and creamy in consistency, which will help it float.
3. Top the glasses up with the green juice so that it forms a separate layer on top and serve with carrot tops and straws.

BEETROOT BERRY SMOOTHIE

Serves 1

Ingredients

1 raw beetroot, peeled and chopped
a handful of raspberries
a handful of strawberries, stalks removed
250ml (1 cup) unsweetened almond milk

1. Whizz all the ingredients together in a blender and serve in a glass with 3 ice cubes.

BLUEBERRY SWIRL

Serves 2

Ingredients

banana
1 ripe banana, peeled
50g (½ cup) rolled oats
2 tbsp almond butter
250ml (1 cup) unsweetened almond milk

blueberry
75g (½ cup) blueberries
1 tbsp chia seeds
2 medjool dates, pitted and roughly chopped

1. Make the banana smoothie first. Whizz all the ingredients together in a blender and pour into two glasses.
2. Next, rinse the blender and whizz all the blueberry ingredients together in a blender with 125ml (¼ cup) water and carefully pour over the banana smoothie, using a spoon to create a swirl on the top.

MANGO PASSION

Serves 1

Ingredients

½ mango, peeled, stoned and roughly chopped
juice of ½ lime
180ml (¾ cup) coconut water
1 passion fruit, seeds and pulp scooped out

1. Add the mango to a blender with the lime juice and coconut water, blend until smooth and pour into a glass.
2. Stir in the passion fruit seeds and serve.

BLACKBERRY CRUMBLE

Serves 1

Ingredients

60g (½ cup) frozen blackberries
1 apple, cored and roughly chopped
2 heaped tbsp rolled oats
250ml (1 cup) unsweetened almond milk
1 tsp baobab powder (optional)
1 tbsp unsalted raw almonds, to serve

1. Whizz all the ingredients except the almonds in a blender until smooth and pour into a glass.
2. Crush the almonds in a pestle and mortar and sprinkle over the smoothie.

Tip ... You can buy blackberries and lots of other berries already frozen, which are great for smoothies.

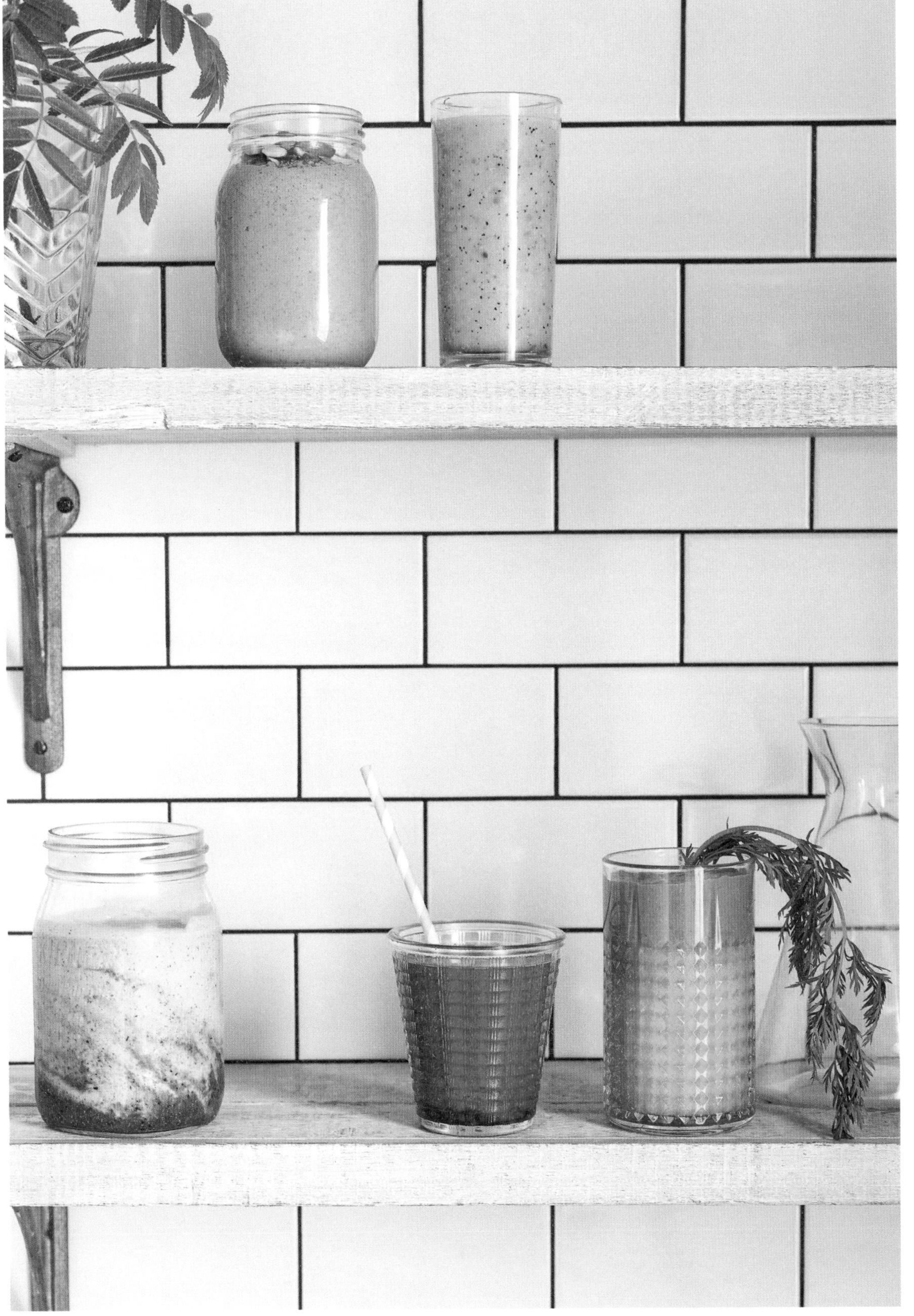

PRE- AND POST-WORKOUT DRINKS

What I drink on workout days hugely impacts my performance and recovery. From a pre-workout drink I need energy and hydration, while after a workout, I want protein to help repair my muscles that have been worked hard.

PRE-WORKOUT

ANTIOXIDANT ENERGY-BOOST SMOOTHIE

Serves 1

Ingredients

1 ripe banana, peeled
1 heaped tbsp rolled oats
40g (¼ cup) blueberries
1 tbsp raw cacao powder
125ml (½ cup) unsweetened almond milk

1. Add all the ingredients to a blender or NutriBullet with 125ml (½ cup) water and blend until smooth.

PEAR + CHIA ENDURANCE JUICE

Serves 1

Ingredients

2 ripe pears, cored and roughly chopped
a large handful of spinach
2 celery sticks
125ml (½ cup) coconut water
1 tbsp chia seeds
1 tsp spirulina powder (optional)

1. Feed the pears, spinach and celery through an extractor juicer.

2. Once the juicer has extracted the pulp, pour in the coconut water and stir in the chia seeds and spirulina, if using.

POST-WORKOUT

PB PROTEIN SMOOTHIE

Serves 1

Ingredients

2 tbsp hemp powder
2 tbsp smooth peanut butter
½ ripe banana, peeled
250ml (1 cup) unsweetened almond milk
¼ x 400g tin chickpeas, drained
1 tbsp raw cacao powder
½ tsp ground cinnamon
1 tsp milled flaxseed (optional)

1. Whizz all the ingredients together in a blender or NutriBullet until smooth.

RECOVERY ROOTS JUICE

Serves 1

Ingredients

6 carrots, peeled and chopped
5cm piece of fresh ginger, peeled
½ tsp turmeric
1 tsp maca powder (optional)

1. Feed the carrots and ginger through an extractor juicer. Once all the pulp has been extracted and you have the juice, stir in the turmeric and maca, if using. Drink soon after juicing.

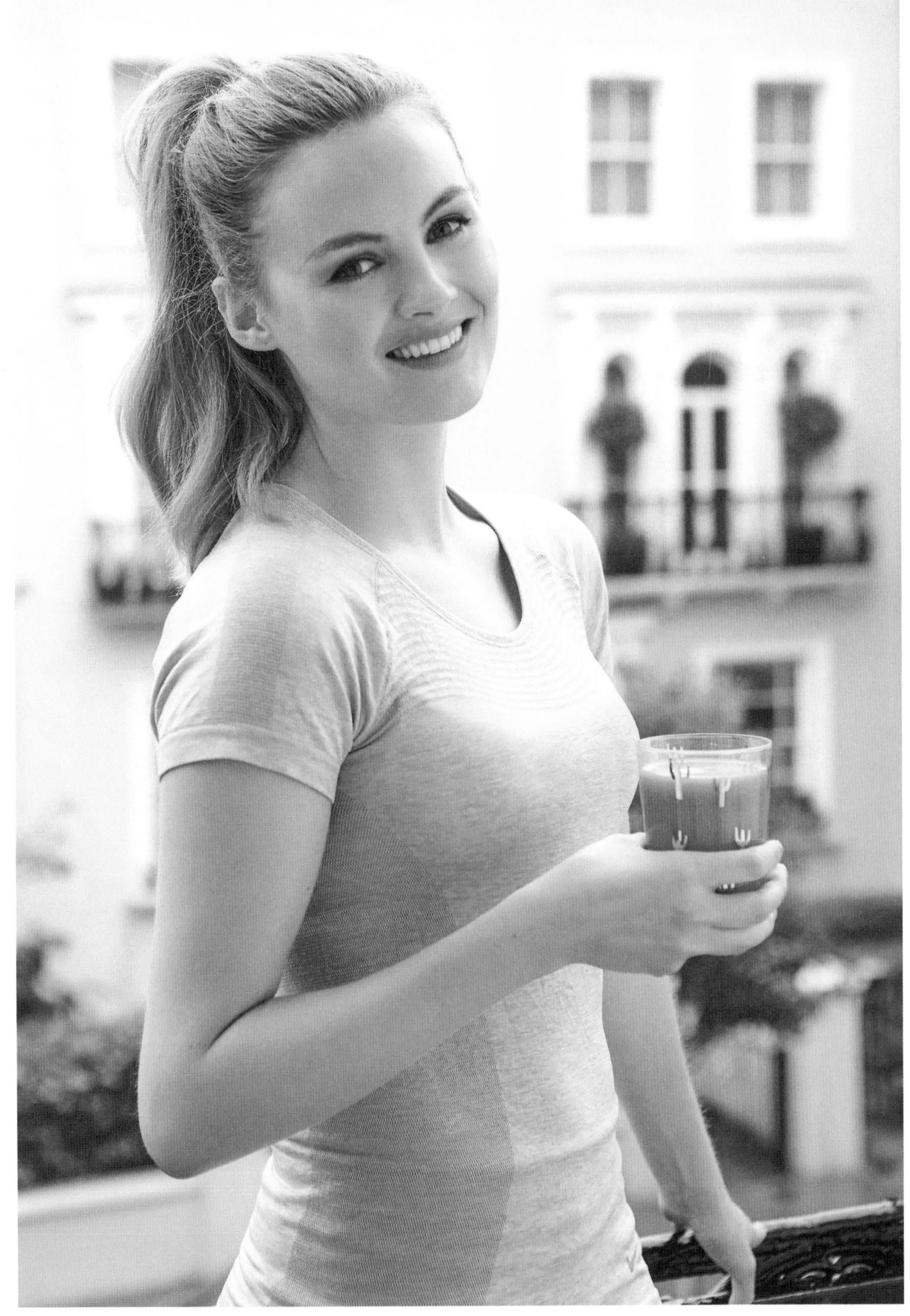

GREEN JUICES – 3 WAYS

Green juices can be a little daunting if you're embarking on a new journey of eating healthier. So I've created three different levels of green juice; sweet for beginners, intermediate with less fruit and more vegetables, and advanced, made from 100% vegetables. All include an abundance of vital vitamins and minerals.

BEGINNER (SWEET + FRUITY)

Serves 1

Ingredients

200g (1 cup) fresh pineapple chunks
5 fresh mint leaves
2 large handfuls of spinach
½ cucumber, chopped
125ml (¼ cup) coconut water

1. Feed the ingredients, except the coconut water, through an extractor juicer.
2. Once the extractor has removed all the pulp, stir in the coconut water.

INTERMEDIATE (COOL + REFRESHING)

Serves 1

Ingredients

125ml (½ cup) coconut water
juice of ½ lemon
1 green apple, cored and roughly chopped
½ cucumber, chopped
½ fennel bulb, trimmed and roughly chopped
2.5cm piece of fresh ginger, peeled

1. Keep the coconut water and lemon aside and feed the remaining ingredients through an extractor juicer.
2. Once the juicer has extracted the pulp, stir in the coconut water and lemon juice.

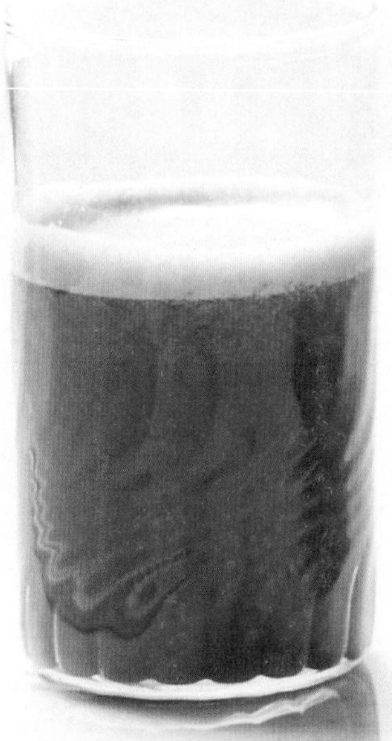

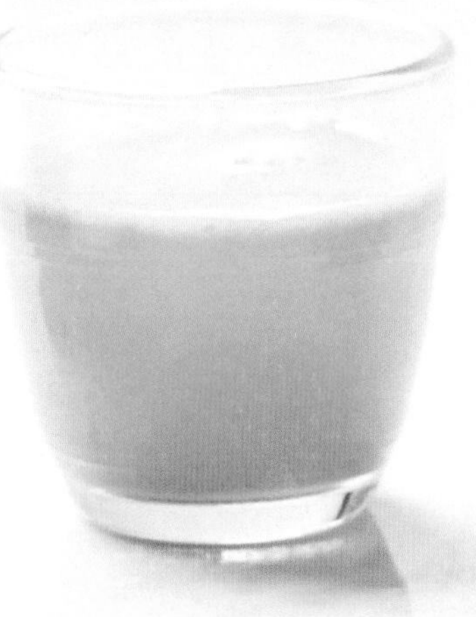

ADVANCED (100% VEG)

Serves 1

Ingredients

½ cucumber, chopped
2 celery sticks, trimmed
2 large handfuls of kale, stalks removed
½ large bunch of fresh parsley, leaves picked
2.5cm piece of fresh ginger, peeled
juice of ½ lemon

1. Gradually feed all the ingredients through an extractor juicer, apart from the lemon juice.
2. Once the juicer has extracted all the pulp, stir in the lemon juice.

Tip ... To get the maximum amount of juice from the kale, spinach and herb leaves, compress them tightly in your hands before adding to the juicer.

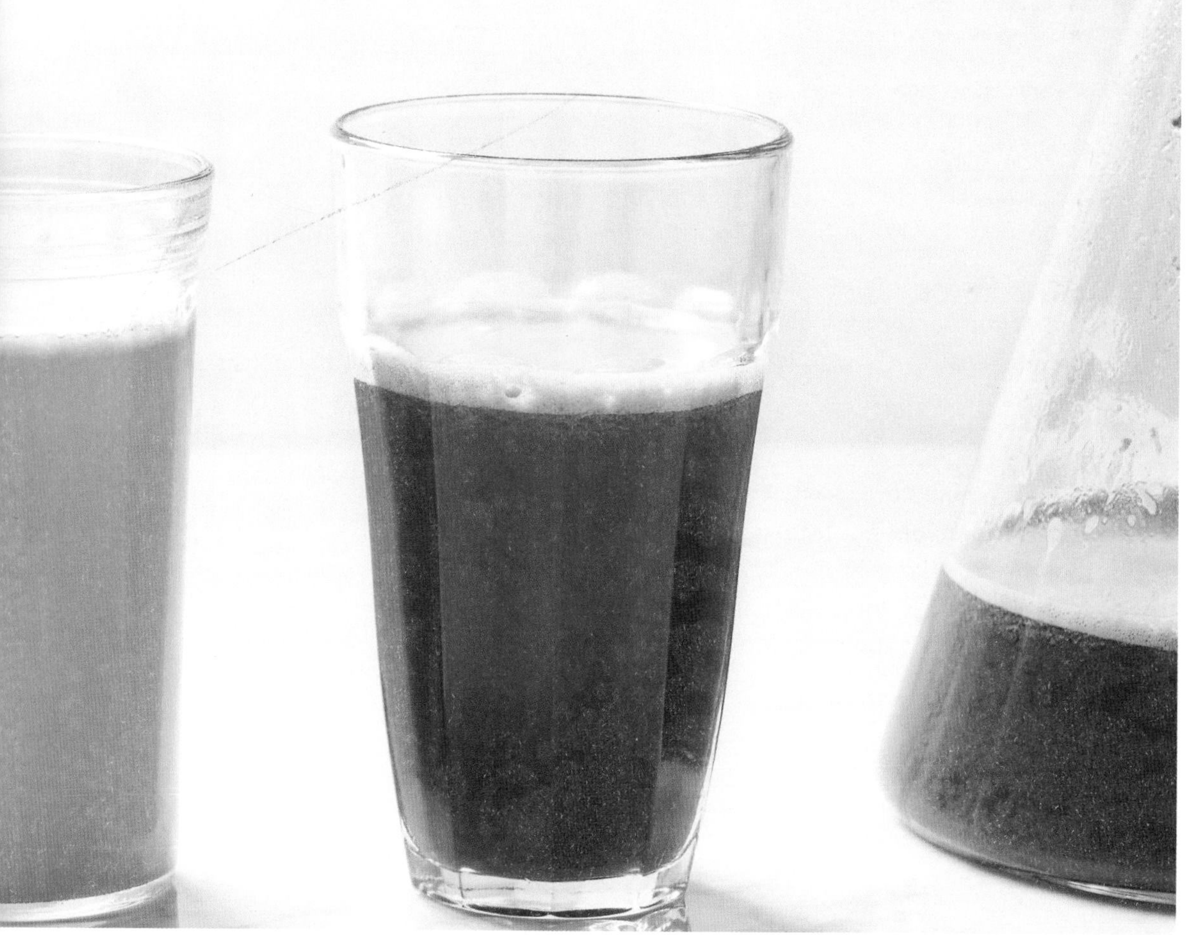

MILKSHAKES – 3 WAYS

Milkshakes are not something I've had to wave goodbye to, as these wonderful naturally sweet ones are, in my opinion, far tastier than any I've ever had from fast-food restaurants. I've made these for friends who are the biggest milk and ice cream fans, who guzzled down my dairy-free versions, licking their lips and asking for more!

CHOCOLATE

Serves 1

Ingredients

250ml (1 cup) unsweetened almond milk
1 frozen banana, peeled and sliced
1 medjool date, pitted and roughly chopped
1 tbsp almond butter
½ tsp ground cinnamon
½ tsp vanilla powder or 1 tsp organic vanilla extract
2 tsp raw cacao powder
25g (¼ cup) unsalted raw walnuts
1 tbsp raw cacao nibs

1. Add all the ingredients, except the walnuts and cacoa nibs, to a blender that works with ice and whizz until smooth.

2. Add the walnuts and cacao nibs and blend just until broken down into small chunks but not totally smooth – we want to keep it chunky but drinkable! Pour into a glass and finish with your choice of toppings.

Topping ideas ...
A teaspoon of goji berries
A teaspoon of raw cacao nibs

VANILLA

Serves 1

Ingredients

250ml (1 cup) unsweetened almond milk
½ tsp vanilla powder or 1 tsp organic vanilla extract
1 parsnip, peeled and chopped
1 tsp barley malt extract
1 tbsp almond butter
1 tsp maple syrup
1 tbsp baobab powder

1. Place all the ingredients into a blender that works with ice, add 2 ice cubes and whizz until smooth.

Tip ... For a smoother consistency, sieve the milkshake before serving or, if you have a juicer, feed the parsnip through an extracting juicer to get the parsnip juice beforehand.

STRAWBERRY

Serves 1

Ingredients

6 large strawberries (about 100g), stalks removed, frozen
1 medjool date, pitted and roughly chopped
½ tsp vanilla powder or 1 tsp organic vanilla extract
250ml (1 cup) unsweetened almond milk

1. Add all the ingredients to a blender that works with ice and whizz until smooth.

Tip ... Feel free to add more strawberries for a stronger flavour.

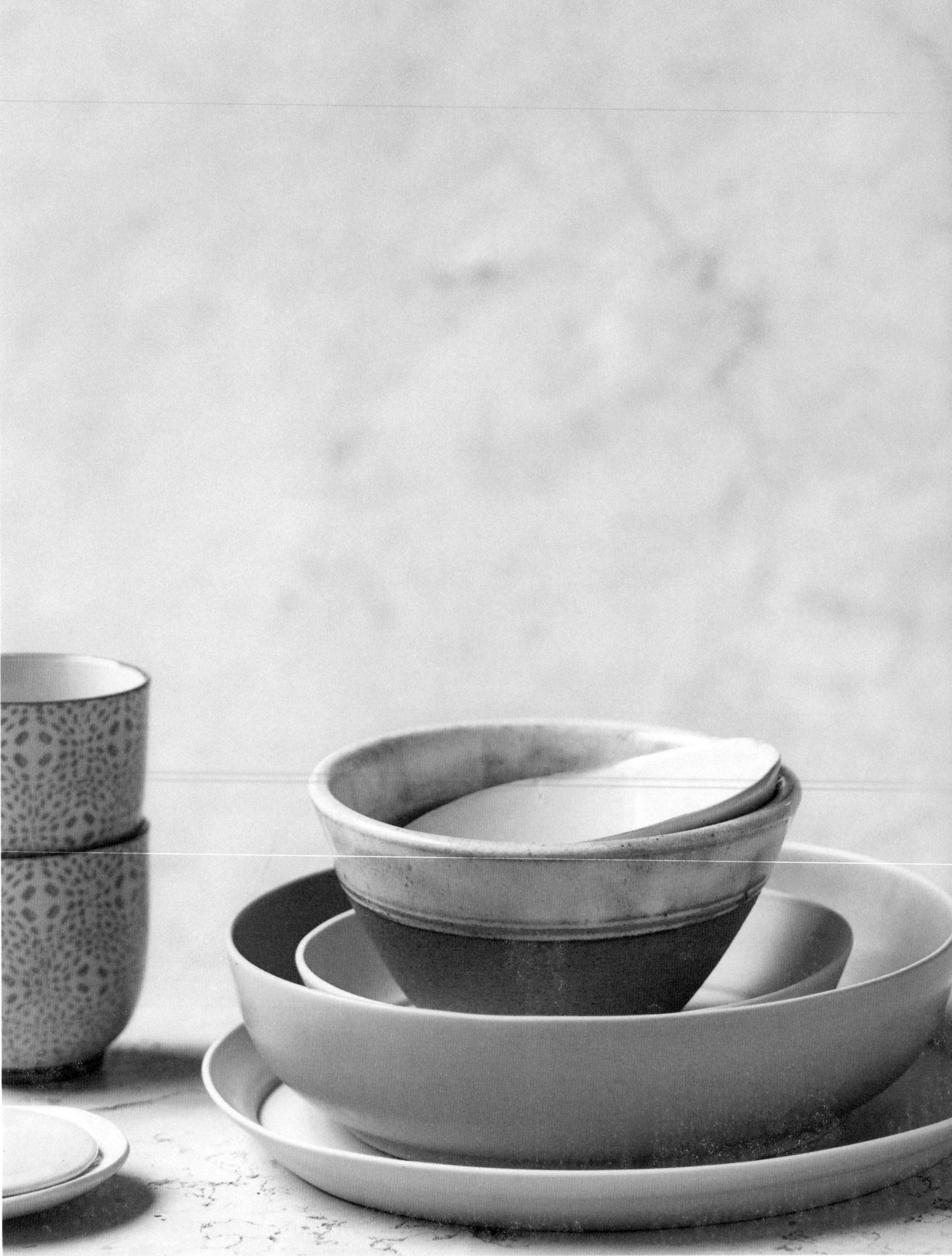

What to eat in a day

What I eat varies depending on what I'm doing. I'm usually running around between meetings, filming and editing videos during the day, then going to events in the evenings. What I eat is also hugely reflective of whether or not I'm doing something active – if I'm going for a run I tend to stick to carb-heavy meals and snacks throughout the day to keep my energy levels high, whereas if I'm strength training I focus on taking in more protein. When I'm not exercising at all, I don't need the extra energy that carbs provide and my body doesn't crave these kinds of foods.

On top of the juices and smoothies that I have listed below, I also drink about 2 litres of water throughout the whole day, every day. It's important to be constantly sipping slowly rather than drinking a whole glass within a couple of minutes! This way you keep your body efficiently hydrated.

WEEKEND
Workout Day

9:30am DRINK/ Morning Detox Water
10:00am BREAKFAST/ Coconut Pancakes with Mango Sauce
11:30am Run
1:00pm AFTERNOON JUICE/ Advanced Green Juice
2:00pm LUNCH/ Roasted Fennel, Lentil + Fig Salad
4:00pm AFTERNOON SNACK/ Root Crisps + Classic Houmous
8:30pm DINNER/ Italian Stuffed Peppers
9:00pm TREAT/ Black Bean Banana Brownies

WEEKEND
Chill Day

10:30am DRINK/ Maple Matcha Latte
12:00pm BRUNCH/ Full English Breakfast
4:00pm AFTERNOON SNACK/ Oat Cakes with Strawberry Chia Jam
8:30pm DINNER/ Squashetti + 'Meatballs'
9:00pm TREAT/ Orange Spiced Cookies

WEEKDAY
Cardio Workout

7:00am BREAKFAST/ Maple Matcha Latte + Banana Bread Porridge
8:00am Run
10:00am POST-WORKOUT SMOOTHIE/ PB Protein Smoothie
1:30pm LUNCH/ Massaged Kale Caesar Salad
4:00pm AFTERNOON SNACK/ Rosemary Crackers with Guacamole
7:30pm DINNER/ Indian Dahl
8:30pm TREAT/ Blueberry Burst Dates

WEEKDAY
Non-Workout

7:30am BREAKFAST/ Mixed Fruit + Nut Granola with unsweetened almond milk + berries
11:00am LATE-MORNING SNACK/ Vanilla Milkshake
1:00pm LUNCH/ Raw Pea + Courgette Soup
3:30pm AFTERNOON SNACK/ Sun-dried Tomato + Cashew Dip with raw carrot and celery sticks
7:30pm DINNER/ Vegetable Laksa

WEEKDAY
Strength Workout

7:00am BREAKFAST/ Antioxidant Energy-Boost Smoothie
8:00am 1-hour gym strength workout
9:30am POST-WORKOUT SNACK/ Raw Fig + Baobab Bar
11:30am MID-MORNING SNACK/ Homemade Oat Cakes with almond butter
1:30pm LUNCH/ Avocado + Turmeric Salad with Quinoa
4:00pm AFTERNOON SNACK/ Supergreen Energy Ball
7:00pm DINNER/ Beetroot Burgers with Spiced Wedges and Summer Salsa

Index

Page numbers in **bold** denote an illustration

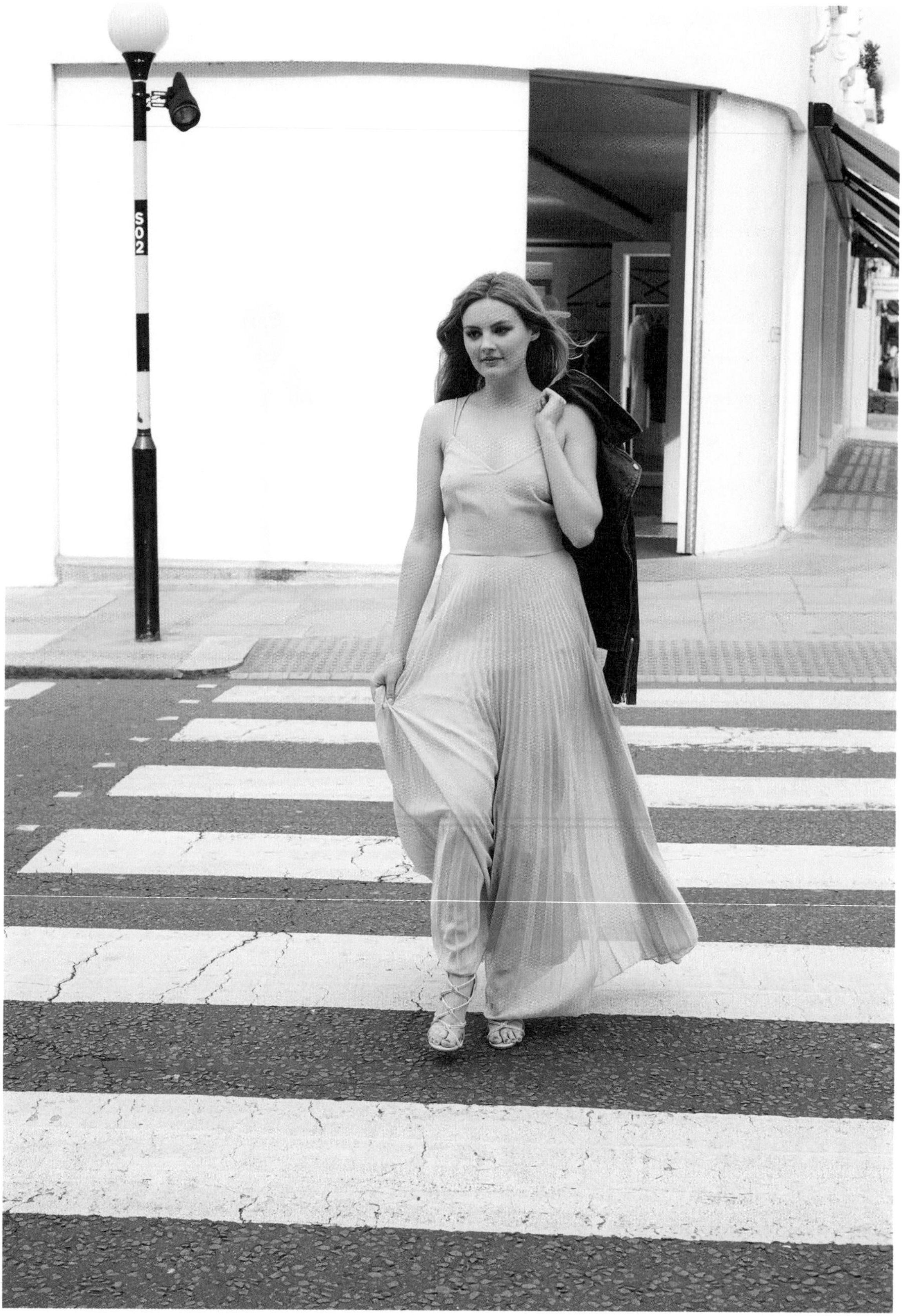

E

F

G

H

I

J

K

L

M

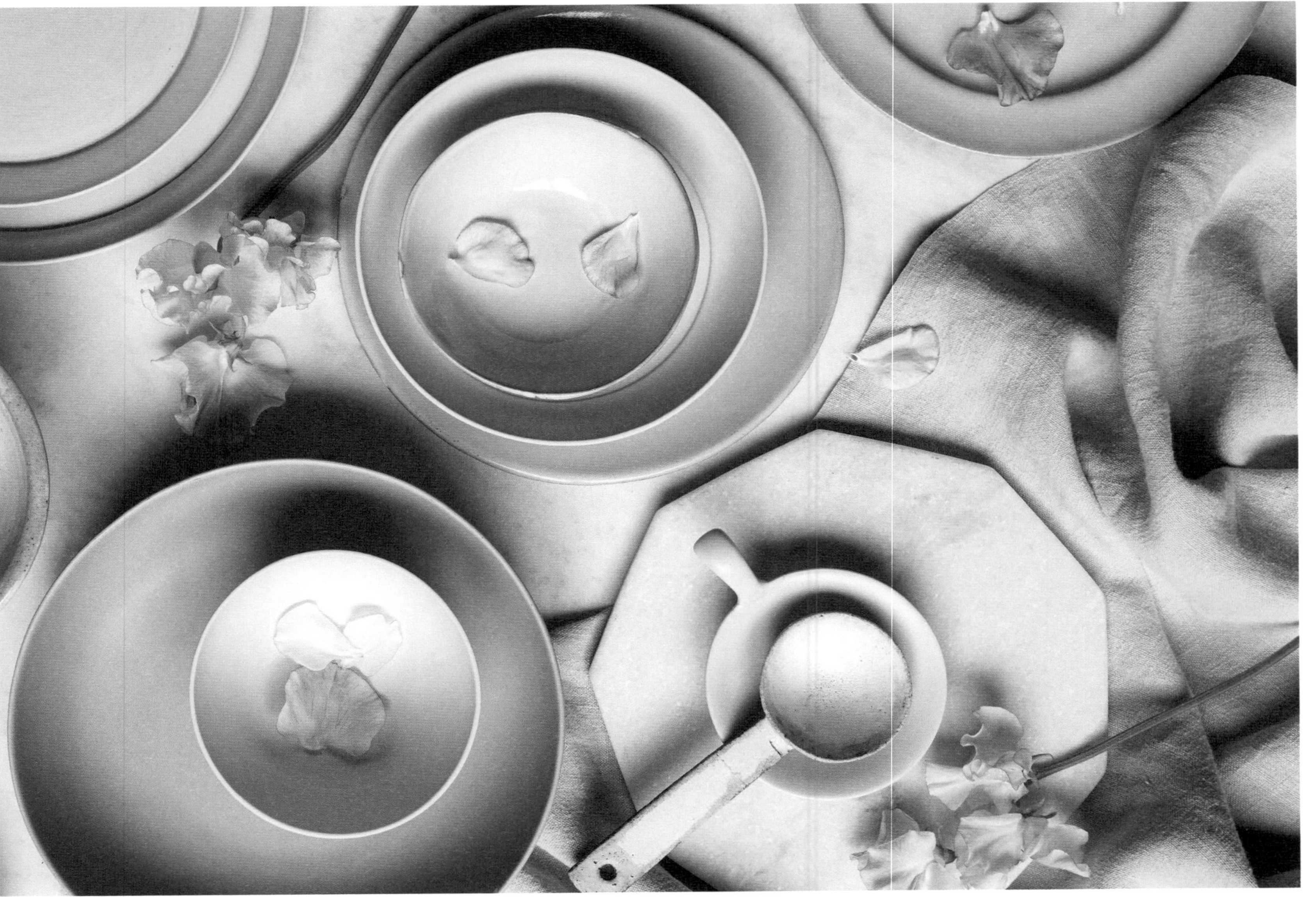

ACKNOWLEDGEMENTS

There are many people in my life who have made this book possible – some who have been there my whole life and some who have only been around a short while but have nonetheless made a huge impact.

I'll start with Gleam, the team that manages me but has become like family over the years. Dom, thank you for having faith in me from the beginning and for seeing through my crazy vision to one day have my very own cookbook, and for helping to turn that into a reality. You've always made me feel like anything is possible. Amy, I really don't know where I'd be without you! Thank you for being there and guiding me through all the incredible projects and opportunities that have emerged over our time working together, and for also being a friend.

Bronagh, thank you for always having a smile on your face and for somehow always being happy! You really do brighten even the most stressful situations. Also thank you to Abigail for being my holy grail on anything book related ... You are the coolest bookworm I know and I appreciate your invaluable knowledge!

Thank you to my wonderful publisher, HarperCollins. Grace, from the day we had our initial meeting I knew you could see my vision of *Eat Smart*. Thank you for listening and for helping me bring it to life. A huge thank you to Isabel, Lucy, Heike and Orlando for all being an absolute pleasure to work with.

Thank you to Tabbi and Alex for spending hours and hours in my kitchen helping me make these recipes and for washing up the mountains of dishes that accumulated in a matter of seconds – you were an absolute godsend and you have no idea how much easier you have made the whole process. Thank you for getting me through it.

My family have always been incredibly supportive of me; whether it's a minor project I'm working on or major life decisions, they're always there. Thank you, Mum, Paul, Grandma, Ian and the rest of my wonderful family. And a special appreciation to my mum for always being at the other end of the phone to give me advice whenever I need her. I love you all so much!

I must also mention Marcus, who has been in my life since we were 11. From your passion for health and fitness to your entrepreneurial focus, you never fail to inspire me. I owe so much of who I am today to you, so thank you.

Thank you to all of the wonderful brands that have supplied the clothes worn throughout the book – Ralph Lauren, ASOS, Sweaty Betty, Marks & Spencer, Dune, Topshop, & Other Stories, Tommy Hilfiger, maje, Keds and Nike.

And finally, thank you to my audience. Frankly, without you this book wouldn't be in your hands – it's all because you subscribe to me, follow me on social media and watch my videos.

My thank you to you is this book, full of recipes that I have put my heart and soul into. I really hope you can tell from making my food how much love has gone into it.

HarperCollins*Publishers*
1 London Bridge Street
London SE1 9GF

www.harpercollins.co.uk

First published by HarperCollins*Publishers* 2016

10 9 8 7 6 5 4 3 2 1

Food styling: Frankie Unsworth
Prop styling: Linda Berlin
Hair and make-up: Frances Done
Clothes styling: Annie Swain

The nutrition and health claims made in this book have all been checked by a registered food nutritionist Mary Lynch. All recipes labelled as healthy have been checked to ensure they are not overly indulgent and that they do contain ingredients with levels of micronutrients that warrant an EU registered nutrition claim. All nutrition claims relating to ingredients themselves have been checked and any health claims made on ingredients have been researched and do not state fact but indicate that this is what the research suggests.

All recipes are based on fan-assisted oven temperatures. If you are using a conventional oven, raise the temperature 20°C higher than stated in recipes.

A catalogue record of this book is available from the British Library.

Main HB ISBN 978-0-00-820380-1

Printed and bound in Spain by Graficas Estella

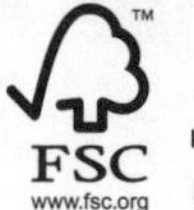

MIX
Paper from responsible sources
FSC™ C007454

FSC™ is a non-profit international organisation established to promote the responsible management of the world's forests. Products carrying the FSC label are independently certified to assure consumers that they come from forests that are managed to meet the social, economic and ecological needs of present and future generations, and other controlled sources.

Find out more about HarperCollins and the environment at
www.harpercollins.co.uk/green

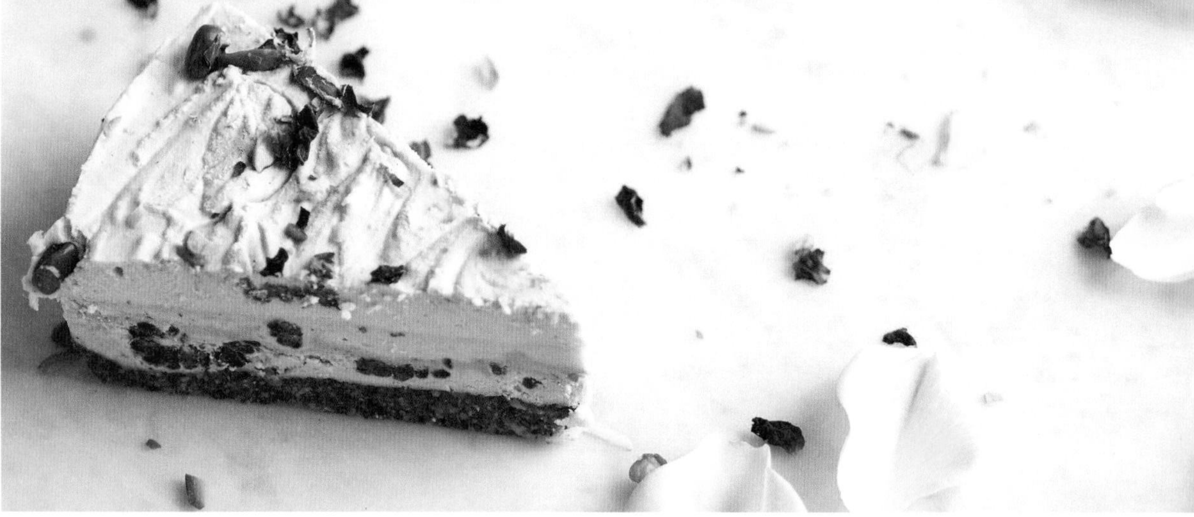